PENGUIN BOOKS

A Walk from the Wild Edge

Jake Tyler is a mental health advocate and adventure athlete. He also works in a coffee shop. *A Walk from the Wild Edge* is his first book.

A Walk from the Wild Edge

JAKE TYLER

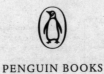

PENGUIN BOOKS

PENGUIN BOOKS

UK | USA | Canada | Ireland | Australia
India | New Zealand | South Africa

Penguin Books is part of the Penguin Random House group of companies
whose addresses can be found at global.penguinrandomhouse.com

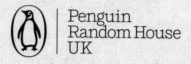

First published by Michael Joseph, 2021
Published in Penguin Books, 2022
001

Typeset by Jouve (UK), Milton Keynes
Printed and bound in Great Britain by Clays Ltd, Elcograf S.p.A.

The authorized representative in the EEA is Penguin Random House Ireland,
Morrison Chambers, 32 Nassau Street, Dublin D02 YH68

A CIP catalogue record for this book is available from the British Library

ISBN: 978-0-241-40117-0

www.greenpenguin.co.uk

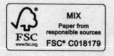

For Mum

The terrain on the upper section of Ben Nevis looked like the surface of the moon – no plants, no grass, no fungi, no life at all; just a vast plain of small grey rocks edging towards the sky. As I perched a thousand metres above the Nevis Forest, breathing plumes of thick mist, I noticed a little white bird that had landed ten yards or so away from me, on a rock in the gap between two precipices. It was a snow bunting. Some people, I'd heard, climbed the mountain just to catch a glimpse of it. It glanced nonchalantly at me, sharing the moment, before it took off and plunged into the dense white cloud between the rocks. In those few seconds of silent appreciation, I realized that I was completely at ease. At ease in my surroundings. At ease in myself. I belonged there, almost as much as the bunting. And as I continued my ascent, the sound of the rocks crunching beneath my boots, my thoughts drifted back to that morning when I'd forgotten that it was possible to feel so alive.

I

March 2016

In just the past month I'd thought of nine or ten ways I could do it. Sticking my head in the oven felt like it would leave the least amount of mess; using a knife would take some serious bottle, more than I felt I had; and while throwing myself in front of a train at Stratford would probably get the job done, the psychological impact on the driver and everyone on the platform was just too awful to think about, and not something I wanted to be responsible for.

I'd been living like a wounded animal for weeks, too hurt to move, begging to be put out of its misery. I longed to eat something I didn't know I was allergic to, to be stabbed in the street, to have an undiagnosed heart condition. But of all the versions of death I could dream up, the one I fantasized about the most was jumping from the room on the fourth storey, above the bar. I imagined standing on the ledge, staring down at a world I didn't understand, a world full of people I didn't feel any sort of kinship with. I imagined a sudden gust of wind, cold and hostile, slapping me across the face, before I took one last breath of dank, polluted London air and released myself, from the ledge and from my rotten, disintegrated life, feeling the briefest rush of terror and adrenaline course through me as I plunged head first towards the pavement.

. . . and then, just like that, it'd all be over. Dreamless sleep forever and ever. No pain, no hate, no sadness. Abrupt, blissful nothingness.

But despite obsessing about death, allowing the image of falling through the air to get clearer and more visceral over time, the thought of killing myself was a desire, not an option. I honestly never thought I'd go through with it – at least, not until that morning.

My shift had ended early. Bethnal Green Road had been quiet, even for a weeknight, resulting in probably the most peaceful evening I'd seen at the Well and Bucket since I'd agreed to take over as manager eight months previously. It was typically a very busy haunt – located off the top of Brick Lane on the fashionable Shoreditch/Bethnal Green border, it was renowned for good food and good, interesting booze, and was tastefully decorated with dark wooden floors, a polished brass bar, and crumbling tiles from Britain's Regency era clinging desperately to the walls. It served as a landmark of sorts, a solid piece of London's social history, and it remained a popular choice with the hordes of young professionals and artisan-spirit purveyors of east London.

After over a decade spent slinging pints and mopping up vomit in Brighton's thriving but slightly mucky bar scene, I had been excited to be asked to oversee a venue with that much class and history. However, only a couple of months in, my initial enthusiasm had begun to fade, and my excitement about landing the 'dream job' was replaced by an intense, rotting feeling inside me that I didn't understand. Something was happening to me. Something was wrong. And what terrified me the most was that I didn't know how to fix it.

That night, after ushering out the last few stragglers, I cashed up and joined my staff for a post-shift drink, slightly earlier than usual. We congregated in our usual spot – on the side of the bar nearest the tiled wall beneath three large Victorian portraits with human skulls superimposed over the faces. I sat there for hours, silently knocking back can after can of half-chilled Camden Hells, half-listening to the usual gossip about customers, friends and current flings, staring at the paintings. They had a macabre quality, and looking at them made me feel closer to death, in a way that was more comfortable than it should have been. I looked towards the ceiling, picturing my room on the fourth floor, and realized that I felt no sense of comfort in doing so.

My bosses hated the idea of me living above the pub, and for good reason. With no clear divide between my job and any sanctuary, I was constantly on high alert and spent most of my time off lying in bed, flinching at every sound that came from the floors below like a dog in a storm. My room was a truthful reflection of how I viewed myself – cold, bare and void of any charm or personality. Waking up in that room every day made me feel like the lowest of the low; lacking even the most basic self-respect to keep it habitable. My hygiene routine had run aground a few weeks previously, and slumping into bed without showering at the end of the night was now a regular thing. Looking into a mirror for longer than a second was starting to torment me, and running my tongue across my teeth felt like licking the felt on an old pub pool table. I was in poor shape, in every conceivable way. And I had never felt so alone.

I thought I had to avoid being found out at all costs and, whenever I felt this way, whenever my mind told me how shit I was, I buried it. I buried it in shallow holes, never deep enough to cover it up completely, so when the working day was over and I was by myself, the feelings re-emerged.

I'd always felt that there were two versions of 'Jake'. Version one is confident, engaged, talkative, has the guts to take on just about anything; version two is quiet, unable to think straight and unsure of who he is. In my mind, V2 posed a constant threat to my more desirable self, V1. V2 was, in my eyes, the most pathetic individual that has ever lived. It's unsettling writing about myself like this – I'd never dream of being so brutal to another human being the way I sometimes am to myself.

I was ashamed of the second version of me, and I carried that shame around with me like a bag of rocks. Surrounded by what I saw to be relentlessly confident people *all* of the time, my lack of consistency was a source of intense embarrassment, and I used so much of my energy trying to hide it. Despite kind of recognizing that hating a side of me was a 'mind' issue, I never once considered that it could be described as a 'mental health' issue. I was convinced that what was going on inside my head was something specific to me, a personality malfunction that was mine to either rectify or ignore as I saw fit. The thought of seeking help from a doctor never even entered my mind. Doctors were for physical ailments – colds, flu, tummy bugs – not for helping with the feeling that there's a crap version of yourself that makes you sad and scared and which constantly threatens the person you want to be.

I sometimes wonder what I'd have done if I'd known I was dealing with depression. Would I have tried to get help earlier? Or would I have been afraid, resisted it, or just not known where to find it?

Night had turned into day, and after finally calling it a night with my staff, I locked the pub and climbed the stairs to my room on the fourth floor. As I lay on my bed, facing the ceiling, a fog swam through and occupied every corner of my mind as the dull London dawn seeped into my bedroom. I spent a few glazed-over moments just staring at the end of the bed. The beer-stained shirt and jeans I'd peeled off lay there, limp and ugly, and I winced, knowing that despite that they were still my cleanest clothes and that I'd have to wear them again today.

Across the room was the window I smoked out of. I used to like sitting there at night, listening to the busy sounds of east London, out of view of everyone on the street below.

As I lay staring at it, sadness engulfing me like bonfire smoke, I realized this was it. The pain I felt was so deep I convinced myself it would be impossible to recover from it. I would never be happy again. In that moment, there was only one way I could see to end the pain.

I focused on the window so intently that everything around it faded to black, and I felt a chill run through my veins. It was over, I knew that. The chill turned into heat and shot so much adrenaline through me I thought I would throw up. In a bid to calm myself before I stood up, I took a breath and began counting down from ten.

Ten . . . nine . . . eight . . . seven . . . six . . . five . . . four . . . *Mum* . . . three . . . *I want my mum* . . .

Somewhere in between unconscious survival instinct and the conscious understanding that my life hung in the balance, I saw her face. Without even thinking about it, I reached for my phone, opened my contacts and found her name: Mum.

Mum is small, like a Hobbit. She lives on a barge that she bought in the Netherlands after she and my dad split up when I was nineteen. She wears woolly socks and drinks hot blackcurrant tea from stained mugs. She has inquisitive blue-green eyes and the same button nose as me. She's named most of the ducks on the River Blackwater in Essex, something she wishes she didn't do because she gets upset when, say, 'Mark E. Duck' goes missing. She once came to my

7

primary school to teach us yoga, and she used to cheer louder than all the other mums at sports day. She meditates every day and burns incense without taking fire precautions. She makes the world's best roast vegetables. She loves watching football, going to gigs and smoking three roll-ups in the evening while she watches *Holby City*. Mum thinks dogs should be dogs and encourages hers, Reggie, to bark at passers-by from the barge wheelhouse. She had a vegetarian food business called Sun and Moon when we were kids and shouted at our childminder after finding out she'd been sneaking me and my brother, Sam, coffee and sausages. She has about a thousand DVDs but doesn't have a favourite film. She is a mother of three, and always made me, Sam and my sister, Frank, feel unconditionally wanted and loved, like we were the centre of her Earth.

'Hello, stinker,' she said. I could almost see her scrunching up her nose, a playful glint in her eye.

A pause. It felt as if my heart was breaking.

'Hi,' I said. Deep, rasping, broken.

'Jake?'

'. . .'

'Are you all right?'

Crying. Breaking. Shattering.

'I don't know what's going on,' I stuttered, my intonation patchy.

Silence.

'I'm really worried . . . I'm going to hurt myself.' I was sobbing.

It's become very common for people to suggest that you 'talk to someone' if you're struggling with your mental health. While this is good advice, sadly it's not always that easy. The pressure to be clear about what's going on in your head and to communicate your pain so that someone else understands

8

is one of the reasons so many people struggle to open up. What you are feeling is disjointed and jarring and nothing makes sense. You feel that no one else could possibly understand, and so you put it off, assuming that if you can't be understood, you can't be helped. What I learned in that moment on the phone with my mum is that opening a door and sharing your mind with another person isn't about seeking answers, it's about no longer being alone in your pain. Letting my mum in somehow made the load lighter. Her love and concern forced their way through the fog, squeezing and weaving, creating a chink of light bright enough for me to see what it was I was considering and to question whether it really was the answer. No doubt about it – that phone call saved my life.

I spent maybe twenty minutes on the phone to my mum, crying mostly, being silent in between. Before she hung up, she gave me a couple of jobs. Number one was to let my employers know what I'd told her. The anxieties I'd been having about being unfit for the role I'd been given, being unable to cope with the stress of management, of there being a hundred other people waiting in line to jump in and do my job, and do it better than me, made the prospect of talking to my employers Mike and Lee – the very people who might confirm that all these things were true – seem a difficult and unnerving assignment. But when I picked up the phone and called Lee, I was met with nothing but genuine concern. It was as if I'd taken the lid off something when I called Mum and it felt a bit easier now to pour myself out. Even though I felt my ability to think clearly and to make decisions was at absolute nil, I still wanted to work. If I left, I would just have more time to obsess about how I was feeling. We decided to reduce my hours to thirty a week, so that day I left the pub by midday, which meant I could tackle the second job Mum had given me – to go and see a doctor. Again, this wasn't something I had previously considered an option, and as a result I had mixed feelings about it – what's the point, what can they do, isn't it just going to be a waste of everyone's time?

Calling the surgery would also mean a hat trick of soul-baring phone conversations before lunch, and that in itself was deeply unsettling. When I called, the receptionist asked me why I needed to see the doctor and, instantly, without pause, the words broke free.

'I think I want to kill myself.'

When I heard those words leave my mouth I felt like I'd revealed a secret I'd sworn never to tell. Fear and panic shot down my arms, my stomach turned over and the blood drained from my face. Saying it had made me think about how close I'd come to dying that morning, and the realization made my skin itch. The breath was knocked out of me by a tidal wave of guilt. Tuesday, 29 March 2016. It could have been a day that everyone who loved me might never recover from, forever tormenting themselves by wondering if they could have done more, why they hadn't noticed something was wrong. I felt sick with shame.

I entered the GP's surgery that afternoon on autopilot. I had no idea what I was going to say, or what would come of the appointment, but it felt right to be doing something, like it was necessary. The doctor sat me down rather than asking me to take a seat and sat next to me, on the same side of the desk. I was numb, a big ball of nothing. He asked what he could do for me and I looked straight into his eyes. They were kind, but in them I could see that he wasn't really sure what to do with me. He looked about my age and was wearing a crisply ironed shirt and trousers pulled tight and unflatteringly around his thighs. After a few moments of awkward silence I started talking, and before I knew it I couldn't stop:

'I nearly killed myself this morning, I think I'm going mad. I'm overwhelmed all the time, I don't even know who I am. I can't remember what feeling happy is like. I've struggled with confidence and low self-esteem for years; I literally hate everything about myself. Sometimes I can pretend to be a different version of me, and people really like him, but I can't do that all the time. I hide everything. I'm deeply insecure. I make people smile because their face is the only thing that can lift me out of the darkness for a moment. I get anxious socially. I can't do my job. I don't sleep properly. I drink every day and take drugs all the time. I don't belong in this world, I'm not like everyone else here. I think I might be crazy. There's this fog inside me and it saturates everything. I can't think straight, I can't articulate myself.'

He listened intently to me tripping over the muddle of words gushing out of me.

It was like with every sentence I was confessing absolute truth, and while it was unbearably uncomfortable and nauseating, it felt like I was doing the right thing. When I finally came up for air something washed over me, encouraging me to fill my lungs and let my jaw unclench. Calmness. Relief. For a few moments, the doctor stared back at me.

After a long pause he asked me a question, the most important question I'd ever been asked:

'Do you actually want to die, Jake, or do you not want to feel like this anymore?'

It was in that doctor's office that I realized I'd become convinced that suicide was what I had to do to free myself of such intense mental pain. I'd not even considered that the two things could be separated. Understanding the distinction between wanting my pain to be over and wanting my life to be over helped me achieve some clarity when my thoughts were at their murkiest, and over the following weeks I kept his question in my mind as I attempted to piece myself back together. I had refused the GP's suggestion that I take a course of antidepressants. I wasn't entirely sure why, but I did. Somehow, I felt that medicating myself wouldn't get to the crux of what was wrong with me. Like the drugs might mask what was really going on. I did agree that seeing a therapist was probably a good idea, so I was given the number of a Cognitive Behavioural Therapist named Irene.

I saw Irene in her eleventh-floor office, far away from the crowded streets nestled below, maybe twice a week for three weeks. I don't remember much of the conversations we had, I only remember that at the time I felt like I was doing something important and necessary by visiting her, and I know that Irene helped change my perspective pretty quickly. She helped me see that my behaviours were simply human behaviours and that what I was doing was exactly what 'we' do in times of trauma. It was interesting to discuss these things, and Irene's insight was often very illuminating. But it didn't do much for how I felt inside. Despite feeling that I now had some support from those around me, I continued to feel withdrawn, lost and jaded, and I was still no closer to 'fixing' the problem.

Depression isn't just misery, it's agony, and carrying it is as exhausting as anything I've ever had to do. A week after that morning where things almost came to a head, it became apparent that I was too ill to work. With a heavy heart and an acute sense of failure, I resigned from my position at the Well and Bucket and ran home.

2

In quitting my job, I might have fled the stress of work, but the weight of what I'd been through was still bearing heavily down on me. I couldn't physically escape it because it wasn't a place or a person or a situation, it was something going on inside me, and in order to escape myself I was going to have to do better than just change postcodes. Being in my home town of Maldon, Essex, felt good, though. The familiarity calmed me. I knew the distinctive smell of mud on the quay when the tide's out; how the tree outside All Saints Church explodes with pink blossom in the spring; how to spot the faint outline of the infamous 'Welcome to Malden' graffiti on the roof of Iceland (the perpetrator calculatingly misspelled 'Maldon' – a sure sign he was from the town and knew just how much it would piss the locals off). Something about being there made me feel close to being reset. It could be something in the estuary air, or how the church bells chime high and musical and carry throughout the town, or seeing the same old faces in the high street – people I've never spoken to but have watched slowly age over time. Maldon is also home to both my parents, both grandmothers, one of my grandads, my uncle, aunt and two of my cousins, so being there feels like I'm being hugged by my entire family. At this point in my life, it's fair to say I was in need of a hug.

My family was a tight unit when I was growing up. My parents had me and my brother, Sam, when they were very young, and when my sister, Frank, came on the scene in 1999 I was already thirteen and becoming my own person. I guess it would make for a good story to say that life was a struggle from the get-go, that the way I felt later in life was the result of a tormented youth and a dysfunctional family, but the truth is I really enjoyed my childhood.

My fondest memories are almost all from the times we spent outdoors as a family. Bundling up in hats, gloves and big, comfy jumpers and driving out to the woods, where Sam and I would chop down bracken and hurtle deep into the trees to 'explore' and 'find clues'. It's the perfect environment to let a kid's curiosity and imagination run wild, opening the door to a world of discovery, freedom and adventure. I held on to those feelings, even after our walks became less frequent as we got older, but I think the escape from reality that nature has always brought me stems from those walks we used to take.

I was proud of my 'outdoorsy' family, even more so when I began to notice how 'indoorsy' a lot of my other friends' families seemed to be – lots of dads in ties, with Sky dishes and microwave dinners; it was a far cry from being brought up by two young hippies. Even after my folks split up when I was nineteen, we all remained close. After selling the family home, Dad got himself a flat above a tanning salon in Maldon High Street, where Sam and I lived until we left home, while Mum went over to the Netherlands, bought herself the barge and brought it back to the quay on the Blackwater estuary, and she's been living in it there with Frank ever since. Maldon's steadily grown into a busy town over the years, and despite being moored near the bustling promenade park ('the prom', as it's known to the locals), Mum's boat *Blackbird* is as peaceful a home as you're likely to find. With Frank at university and Dad having moved into a smaller place, I decided it would be there, with Mum, that I'd go to get better.

I quickly became the key feature in Mum's living room – a fifteen-by-twelve-foot cabin with dark wooden panelling on the walls, a small log burner on the far wall, opposite the comfiest battered red sofa in the world, and a colourful rug, acquired on one of Mum's many trips to India, covering the entire floor. Hanging on the walls and windowsills are a number of framed pictures and trinkets, including a few Buddhist monuments and an old Bob Dylan fly poster. It's a far cry from the squalid, desolate walls in my room in Shoreditch. Next to the TV hangs a sign that reads, 'What would Elvis do?' – kind of apt, I thought, as I lay there for days on end, comfort-eating sweets and crisps and crumpets and chips, indulging in short-term pleasure at the expense of long-term happiness.

After a week or so on the boat my days were beginning to blur into each other. With no job, no fixed routine and no energy, my only tasks were to get out of bed in the morning and go back to bed at night. I found myself staring at the space between me and the TV, letting insurance adverts and the canned laughter from various sitcom reruns wash over me until it was time to go to bed. I didn't even know what interested me anymore, what my opinions were or what gave me pleasure. Funny programmes didn't make me laugh; the news didn't make me angry. Every time Mum spoke to me I felt like crying, and every time she hugged me I felt nothing. Before she went to work most days she would suggest something for me to do – go for a walk, have a shower, write my feelings down – and every evening when she got home I felt like I was disappointing her for not having attempted any of it. She never acted disappointed, of course, but that didn't stop the guilt. I felt like I'd eventually break her spirit just by being near her, and that upset me more than anything. I'd never felt more lost or more unsure of who I was. I truly believed that there would be no way to fully recover from what was happening to me and, what was worse, I didn't even care. As long as I had my duvet, there was a part of me that, in a way, was prepared to be this person forever, because, although I felt sad, it was kind of comfy and required the least amount of effort. Depression's very good at pulling you into a hole and hugging you while you're down there. The desire to get better is replaced by a type of comfort that becomes, strangely, your mind's only source of pleasure, and over time that feeling of comfort becomes addictive. I took some sort of weird satisfaction in not having to consider whether I was making the right choices, whether I was looking out for my future self, whether I was ever going to get on the property ladder, whether my friends liked me.

A few more weeks passed before the urge to help myself surfaced. It was little more than a faint silhouette on the horizon, small and far away but there nonetheless, slowly heading towards me. I started to feel the need to do something with my days so I didn't feel like a slave to my emotions, something that made me feel like I was running myself rather than depression running me. And so, on the millionth time of Mum suggesting I take Reggie out for a walk, I eventually said yes.

The air outside was warm, but there was a slight chill from the wind, and Reggie and I walked beside the river, stopping occasionally to inspect the ducks. This soon became my and Reggie's daily routine. On our first few outings I didn't venture too far from the safety of the boat, but after a week or so I decided a change of scenery might be nice, so we took a walk across town to 'Leech's' – a humble and well-cared-for memorial garden that gazes over the tops of the trees of the town's neighbouring woodland and was the setting for many of my childhood memories. It was where my parents told me and my brother that they were expecting my little sister, and where I was introduced to the wonders of cannabis by an older kid who got me so high that I ended my first drug experience greening out (as was the expression) in my bedroom with the curtains drawn against the sun, while playing *Doom*. Leech's was also where my neighbour and I once discovered a fledgling starling and spent the whole afternoon 'teaching it to fly'; we charged up and down the field holding the tiny bird gently between our fingers, moving our hands like the conductor of an orchestra to encourage it to flap its wings. After hours of 'training' and several nosedives, my neighbour let the bird go and the two of us cheered as we watched it soar over the bushes at the end of the garden and fly away to begin its life (we hoped).

My walks were turning into a daily dose of nostalgia, and with every day I looked forward to them more and more, and the more I was seeing positive change in myself. I noticed that my posture was improving each time I stepped off the boat, a sign that my confidence was returning, and on our morning strolls along the river I often found myself in a state of quiet appreciation of the stillness of it and the beautiful simplicity of nature. Some mornings the water looked so calm it was almost hypnotic, and as I stared into the mirrored image of the blue-and-yellow sky and every bird that flew over it, a peace would settle within me, a feeling that, not so long before, I wasn't sure I'd ever be able to experience again. Moments like these were occurring more frequently, and the serenity I felt in them began to spill over into the rest of the days. My duvet was seeing less and less daytime action, I was washing my clothes, my sleep was falling into a more normal pattern – even my hot-cross-bun intake was beginning to waver. I had begun thinking about what meals I'd like to eat and buying ingredients – avocados for guacamole, potatoes for sausage and mash – rather than just sloping off to Costcutters for a frozen pizza and a bag of Big Hoops. I started responding to messages and even initiated the occasional chat with friends I felt I hadn't checked in with for a while. I was beginning to feel like me again, version one – the version I like – the Jake who looks after himself, and does things.

One grey afternoon in Leech's garden I freed Reg from her lead and watched her bound towards the trees, as she always did. But today she was distracted by a fly or a bee and chased it determinedly. After she'd snapped wildly a few times at thin air, charging clumsily towards it, I found myself beginning to laugh. Not in the desperate, false way I had been for the benefit of other people over the past however long but a genuine just-for-me explosion of laughter. It was the first time I'd laughed properly in months. I felt a warmth flow through me, the same kind of warmth I now feel after a run, or when my gran (Mum's mum) waves me off from her front door after a visit. Real, fluttery, but solid, a glow that spreads through my whole body. I sat calmly for a moment, not looking forwards or backwards, not focusing on who I was or my place in the world, just sitting on a bench, Reggie resting trustfully against me. I was enjoying the awareness of being there and, most importantly, feeling like I belonged there – a sensation I welcomed wholeheartedly after months and months of feeling like an uninvited guest in every setting I found myself in.

I was comfortable in the silence, involved in my surroundings and free of unwanted noise or concern, and I realized something – I felt good. The colours around me were vibrant, the loyal and affectionate energy between Reggie and me was real, and my body, the body I sat there in, the body I had so nearly destroyed a month or so previously, was alive and functioning and capable of so much. I began thinking about how I'd got here, to this point where I now felt good, puzzling over how I'd managed to hoist myself out of such a deep, vast blackness into a place that now shone with optimism. I thought about Mum, how after I'd reached out for her she'd pulled me out from the bottom of something, and about being home, how the familiarity of the town had made me remember who I was. I thought about Reggie, how our walks had given me something to do, how her company got me off the boat and out into the open. And nature – I realized how healing simply being outside had been for me, being mindful of the warmth from the sun, the coolness of the air; how watching the trees dance in the wind and the river reflecting the sky seemed to stop time. I was remembering how at home I'd always felt in the outdoors as a kid, never, ever ready to go home, never fussed by rain and cold. I realized that I had starved myself of something I'd never known was so essential to my well-being, something I now understood I had to relearn. Being outside wasn't just about fresh air and earthy smells, it had given me the mental space I needed to let go of poisonous thoughts, to recognize that, as insufferably painful as my life had become, I had never actually wanted to die, I had just needed to remember what it was like to feel alive.

Something else was happening, too, something unexpected – an idea, or at least the beginning of an idea. With my mind alive and buzzing, I clipped Reggie's lead on and headed back into town. I tied Reggie up outside a bookshop and went inside, scouring the shelves until I spotted what I was after – a map of Great Britain. As I paid at the counter, I briefly wondered if anyone had ever been so excited to buy a map of their home country.

Back on the boat, I kicked my trainers off, opened the

map and spread it out flat on Mum's living-room rug. I grabbed a Sharpie from the drawer under the kitchen table and began furiously circling every section of natural Britain I could see – national parks, AONB (areas of outstanding natural beauty), trails, beaches – anywhere that was green and didn't have tangles of roads coming out of it. I vanished into a nomadic daydream, picturing myself walking through pure British countryside with just a bag on my back, my skin tanned and my hair bleached by the sun. I saw myself hiking through the Lake District, the Scottish Highlands, along the rugged coast of Cornwall. And in doing so, I found myself wondering . . .

How had I let it go so wrong? What had I been doing all this time, allowing myself to be restricted, to stay in one place for so long and let that place eat me up? Somewhere along the line I'd lost touch with the boy who loved disappearing into the woods to cut down bracken. I'd been conforming, trying to live a life that made sense to other people, working myself into sickness, trying to combat negative feelings by buying stuff I didn't need. My life hadn't been especially difficult, I just hadn't given myself a chance. I hadn't paused to see where I was headed, I hadn't looked out for myself, and I hadn't fed my soul anything real in a long, long time. I felt the simultaneous need to escape but also to gain control.

I looked down at my map. Chaos. Frenzied notes and broken circles fought one another for space on the page. But my mind was clear – something felt right. Within the mess, I scouted for possible places to walk, beautiful areas to explore where I could reconnect with a world I so desperately wanted to feel again – the natural world. There were so many places to go. I couldn't decide between them, so in the end I connected all the circles I'd drawn with a thick, black line. What appeared before me was a giant loop. A lap of Great Britain.

I stared at it for a few minutes, letting my mind get high on daydreams about living life as a drifter. Walking for days and weeks on end, immersed in idyllic surroundings with no material possessions and not a care in the world. A life where breathing lungfuls of untarnished air and watching the landscape transform from coast to forest, from hills to mountains, became my routine. I imagined the privilege of watching the sun rise and fall in a new setting every day, the bliss of sleeping under a canopy of stars and, finally, I pictured myself standing at the top of a mountain, nothing but beautiful open space expanding for miles and miles beneath my feet in every direction.

I thought about the concept of triumph over adversity, how hitting rock bottom is what some people must have to do to unlock their potential. I was fresh out of my lowest point, where I felt like I had nothing, and so, in a way, I was back at zero again. Nothing to lose, no expectations, no plans. This was a chance for a new everything, a life that I wrote out myself, that started with me simply leaving. I needed to just go. I wasn't walking away from anything; it felt more like I was walking towards something. Perhaps it was the massiveness of my collapse, but I couldn't help but think big. I knew, in that moment, that I was going to walk a lap of Great Britain and rediscover just how incredible life could be.

3

I've come to realize that stepping away from everything for a short time when you're feeling overwhelmed by it can actually be the most productive thing you can do. Having head space is crucial to working out exactly what it is that needs to change. If you can identify the things that need to change, then do yourself a huge favour and change them. If you can't change the situation, try and change how you approach it or look at it. Once life becomes manageable, it stops being so overwhelming. And there's one thing that's certain: no one fantasizes about driving full speed away from a life they're enjoying.

Standing there, astride my map in Mum's living room, I began to walk the route in my mind. It began in Brighton, the city I'd lived in for eight years before I moved to east London and a place I still considered my home from home. From Brighton's Palace Pier, the path went west in more or less a straight line, hugging the three hundred or so miles of coastline that connects the coastal counties of southern England – Sussex, Hampshire, Dorset, Devon and Cornwall. At Britain's most south-westerly point, Land's End, the line continued along about four hundred miles of coast to Bristol, passing through Exmoor National Park in North Devon, as well as the counties of Somerset and Gloucestershire. After a loop of around seven hundred miles around Wales (my black line passing without pause through the Brecon Beacons, the Pembrokeshire Coast and the epic mountains of Snowdonia), the route shifted east into the English Midlands, then swung north for roughly two hundred miles along the Pennine Way, which cuts through both the Peak District and Yorkshire Dales national parks.

I thought for a moment about the possibility of making my journey public, of the hope it might bring to others. By showcasing Britain's most stunning natural areas I might inspire other people to get outside to experience the healing power of nature for themselves. I felt so caught up in my idea it was like all the answers to everything we spend our whole lives looking for were right there, just outside our front doors. Hugging my arms around myself to slow my heart, I squeezed my eyes shut and let the sun beaming through the window bathe my face. When I opened my eyes again, I continued tracing the line to Cumbria, in the Lake District. How many miles had my finger covered to get there? After a quick tot-up, it was around the 1,200-mile mark. I had my first moment of hesitation. Maybe this was all a bit much.

As I followed the eighty-four-mile section of Hadrian's Wall, beginning at Bowness-on-Solway, the magnitude of what was involved in doing a 'lap of Britain' began to dawn on me. This was nuts. No one was going to take me seriously when I told them I was going to attempt this. But, for some reason, that only made the prospect of doing it more appealing. Imagine if I pulled this off – an overweight, clinically depressed barman with flat feet and a coke habit. The idea was so potent and all-consuming I decided to stop thinking about whether it was possible and began simply believing that I would succeed. This level of self-belief would have been unusual enough for me on a good day; the fact that I had this much confidence while I was still in the (albeit loosening) grip of depression was nothing short of a miracle.

I ran my finger up the coastal path of the English north-west before crossing the border and entering the section of Britain that excited me the most. Scotland. My route into

Scotland again followed the coastline, north for roughly 150 miles to Edinburgh, then across to Glasgow and north again along the famous West Highland Way, ninety-six miles of lochs and mountains to Fort William. From there, I traced seventy-nine miles along the Great Glen Way, hugging the banks of Loch Ness, to Inverness. After that it was just a thousand miles or so south through the Cairngorms, the south-east coast of Scotland, the North York Moors, the east of England, East Anglia, Essex, London, and then – bosh, back at the Palace Pier for a cup of beer and a bag of hot doughnuts.

Looking at the map felt like looking into my future, but it didn't feel real, more like I'd just cast myself in the lead role of an epic adventure story. This would be a once-in-a-lifetime voyage for anyone, and so, with no prior experience and no real business putting myself forward for such a colossally impractical venture, I simply thought, fuck it. And started planning.

I kept my plan to myself for about a week, letting it fine-tune itself in my head before I told my mum, who has a history of bringing my more, let's say, 'romantic' projects back down to earth. Once, when I was nineteen, I got it in my head that out of all the directions my life could go in after college, moving to Nepal to train with Tibetan monks was the stand-out vocational choice. My propensity for big, unrealistic ideas and Mum's sensible outlook has kept me grounded over the years, so I was a little worried about how she'd react to this one. A grandiose venture like walking a lap of the UK was, in all probability, just as shoot-down-able as a monastic life up a Nepalese mountain, so before I let the cat out of the bag I had to make doubly sure I'd thought it all through properly.

To my surprise, when I did tell her, my idea was met with little more than a raised-eyebrow smile. No laughter, no eye-rolling and no immediate questions. If anything, Mum seemed happy that I appeared so animated after months of despondency, and even indulged me when the plan started developing with small comments like 'I've always wanted to go up to the Highlands' and, when I was researching backpacks, 'Which one's going to be your Doritos pocket?'

Mum's got a real talent for questioning my reasons for doing things without pushing me one way or the other, balancing any serious questions with a genuine interest in my life. Her concern is never intrusive; she encourages me to make my own mistakes, only taking the piss when I'm saying something really stupid – and even this is done with so much love I could never get annoyed by it. The night we sat down together to talk through my plans she treated the conversation as if I were coming to her for advice on applying for a new job, or buying a car, welcoming my ideas as real life decisions and not just the ramblings of a jobless dreamer. The scent of Mum's blackcurrant tea filled the space between us and, her arms enveloping her knees, she leaned forward and fixed her eyes on mine and smiled.

'Right, go on, then,' she said.

'Right, so.' I crushed my cigarette out in the ornate tiled dish in the centre of the table and wondered briefly if I should quit smoking. 'All right, let's forget the actual walking bit for a minute,' I said. 'I want to tell you why I'm doing this.'

She raised her head, her expression turning to one of curiosity.

I clasped my hands together. 'I didn't know how I was going to get better after what happened to me in London,' I started.

Mum dipped her head slightly to acknowledge my pain without breaking my flow.

I brushed my thumb back and forth across my knuckles and continued. 'I really didn't think I was ever going to get better, you know. I couldn't see a way out. But taking Reg for walks, it's the missing link connecting me back to a bit of me I didn't even know had gone missing. I haven't had anything else, I haven't taken one antidepressant, haven't gone to any more therapy sessions. The space and fresh air and walking have made me feel like this. I don't know where it's come from. But something's telling me this is something I have to do. There's nothing to hold me back right now, but who knows how long that'll last. This is my chance to do something.'

I was struck by the similarity between this conversation and the one I'd had just a few months ago with the tight-trousered doctor. My mind was again overflowing with emotion that I couldn't really understand or process, only this time it wasn't devastating, it was heartening. This time, the breaths that followed the tumbling words were delicious, full of possibility, powerful. Hearing those words spoken in my voice excited me. I knew then that I was going to get better, and this was how I was going to do it.

Mum nodded. 'This is what you've needed, Jakey, something to throw yourself into, and it probably doesn't get more nourishing or wholesome than living outdoors for six months. And you're really sure that this is the thing that's going to make you feel better?'

'Yeah, I know it will.'

'Well,' she said, 'you'd better get on with it then.'

At this stage I was excited, and that was about it. I hadn't thought about the actual walking, my safety, my poor fitness levels or whether I'd make a plan. Jake version one was happily taking the lead, in his classic 'Act now, think later' way. I wasn't sure of any way to reach other people than to share what I was planning to do on my social media – through words. I wrote a short piece a bit like a mission statement that I thought could act as my shop window:

Today, film, journalism and social media can be used to spread aware-ness, and I'm happy to see the complexities and hardship of mental illness filter more into collective thought than ever before. People affected by conditions such as depression and anxiety have a chance to connect with other sufferers on global platforms, become inspired to make change and support those who are desperate to get well but are too afraid to open up. I believe inspiration to be the first step in learning how to manage mental health, and I'm about to embark on an adven-ture that I hope will inspire people to take control and live the life they want to live.

My name's Jake Tyler. I'm thirty years old and I live with depres-sion and anxiety. In March this year I fell deep into the darkest state of mind that I've ever experienced. I was consumed by relentless thoughts of helplessness, isolation and even suicide and the pain I felt was unbear-able. Something had to change. After a lot of time spent researching and disregarding various medical options, I decided to focus on my physical health. Long walks and fresh air helped clear my head and helped me appreciate the beauty of nature that is right here on my doorstep. I was able to dig myself out of a hole, and this got me thinking.

Why don't more people do this? How can something as simple as taking a walk and encountering the natural beauty of this country make me feel this much better?

My plan is to walk around Great Britain, covering every national park, to show people that there is beauty nearby, no matter where on this island you live. There's a way to get exercise and fresh air that is enriching, life-affirming and, crucially, a perfect way to clear your head and take steps towards recovery.

Writing this wasn't easy. There was a lot of deleting and rewriting, editing and pacing around Mum's living room. I was exposing the side of me that I had purposely and strategically hidden throughout my life. My friends and family were going to know that I had wanted to die. I wondered whether there would be judgement, people asking how someone who had a pretty nice life on paper could be so unhappy, questioning what was wrong with me and why I couldn't just be happy. Whether, now they would see the real me, they would feel deceived because I had been pretending to be someone else for so long. I sensed that this would be the start of many uncomfortable and revealing conversations. Without giving myself long enough to talk myself out of it, I pressed 'post' and threw my phone under the sofa cushions. Something about revealing my vulnerable side so publicly made me want to throw up.

We all like to pretend that we do what we want and we don't care much for the opinions of others, but we do. We all want to be accepted. We all want to be considered 'normal' (whatever the hell that means). I knew that this would be an easier undertaking if I had support. After a few minutes pacing anxiously around the boat, I grabbed my phone and unlocked my screen to find something beautifully unexpected – messages from friends offering support and kind words, responses from family expressing pride and encouragement. People I hadn't spoken to in years all of a sudden seemed prepared to share their most personal thoughts with me, while some people in my life who seemed so together, so confident and uninhibited, were uniting with me through messages of solidarity, revealing that they, too, had been struggling to manage their lives and minds. It was overwhelming. I'd felt so separate for so long and, now, through finally being honest with myself and daring to voice my feelings, I felt more connected than ever to the people in my life, past and present. It upset me, too, though; the lid had been well and truly blown off, and inside it looked like nearly everyone was struggling, and some had found themselves in a place as dark as the one I had been in. For a moment I felt relief, even happiness, that it wasn't just me. There were other people who knew what it was like to be overwhelmed by sadness and despair, people who had also experienced thoughts of suicide, friends who felt like they had different versions of themselves, family who hadn't known where to go for help. Something bigger than I had imagined was going on: it appeared life was proving to be too difficult for everyone. How strange that none of us felt comfortable talking to each other about it.

With my route planned and the idea well and truly out there, the only thing left to think about was what I was going to take with me. As well as walking every day, I would have to camp, so the next thing on the list was researching kit: clothing, camping equipment, medical supplies and maps. I trawled through endless forums and reviews, scribbling notes frantically, weighing up the benefits and necessity of an item against carrying it on my back every day. In the end, I settled on the following:

1 × Wild Country Zephyros 2 tent
1 × 2/3 season sleeping bag
1 × 60–70-litre rucksack
1 × pair top-quality walking boots
5 × pairs double-layered hiking socks
1 × weatherproof jacket
1 × lightweight waterproof jacket
2 × base-layer tops
2 × mid-layer tops
1 × fleece

1 × pair of weatherproof gloves
1 × pair of hiking trousers that zip off at the knee and
   become hiking shorts (sexy)
1 × dry bag
1 × first-aid kit
1 × head torch
2 × 1-litre aluminium water bottles
1 × power bank
Total cost = approx. £900

Since I didn't know what berries I could safely eat or how to set a rabbit snare, I realized I'd also need a bit more money than I had. It was difficult to gauge even roughly how much I'd need to cover me while I had no other source of income. I made incredibly vague estimations about what distance I would manage each day, trying to take into account terrain, elevation, weather and the odd day of rest. Through the wonders of modern technology (Google Maps), I worked out that my route around Britain was in the region of three thousand miles, which meant that, by my calculations, by walking a half-marathon distance (thirteen miles) every day, it would take me roughly seven months to complete my 'lap'. I figured a safe daily budget of £20 should be enough to sustain me in carbohydrates and protein-dense food and cover the occasional hostel bunk when camping wasn't an option, and any other unforeseen expenses. This gave a total cost of £4,260, plus the £900 for outdoorsy supplies, so minus the £1,000 or so I had to my name at the time, I needed to acquire just over £4,000 to make it all possible. To raise that amount with no source of income, I would basically need everyone I knew to chip in, as well as quite a few strangers. It didn't feel great, asking for money to make my adventure possible, but people seemed happy to give, knowing it would ultimately create a platform to spread awareness on an important issue. The walk would also facilitate a seven-month fundraising period for an at that stage unconfirmed mental-health charity.

It felt ambitious, but I had a good feeling about it. Something about the sequence of events: me putting the vulnerable hidden me (Jake V2) out there, the intrigue and appeal of a journey of self-discovery, the urge to inspire other people to take their own mental health into their own hands – it all seemed to resonate with people. People believed in it, so everyone chipped in. Within three weeks, the total had been raised and, by the end of the allotted time for crowd-funding, 'Take a Walk' (as I had temporarily branded the challenge) had amassed a total of £4,232. I was dumbfounded. This mad idea I'd had that came to me while I was out walking Reggie, an idea that may as well have fallen from the sky, and in the wake of the most painfully miserable time in my life, had become real – and through the immense generosity of everyone who pledged, including my former bosses Mike and Lee, it was game on.

4

People have bold, ambitious fantasies about what they could do with their lives all the time. When I wasn't daydreaming about becoming a Tibetan monk, I envisioned myself in all types of exciting scenarios, living all types of exciting lives – buying a van and driving through America, learning to paint so I could make huge portraits of my favourite people and, more recently, traversing the coast of Iceland. The main reason we tend not to just go for it is because ideas that deviate from 'finish school, get a job, find a partner, buy a house' can be so easily disregarded as fanciful, and we all have a tendency to bring ourselves back down to earth when an idea gets 'too big'. For me, though, this time it felt different. Emotion and meaning were driving it, and I couldn't give myself even a window of time to opt out. So, from the day I sat in Mum's living room scribbling on that map, I gave myself two months. Two months to plan it all and get all the stuff I needed, two months to do sit-ups and press-ups and walk long distances daily, and to stop eating a pack of doughnuts a day. I set 26 June as my leaving date, three months from when I felt sure I was going to end my own life. With some residual cravings for booze and drugs, and buffalo sauce still down the front of one of my jumpers, I acknowledged that giving myself as little as two months to get match fit was pushing it, but I reasoned I would get progressively fitter the more miles I walked. The impact of walking Reggie for a couple of hours every day was fairly instant. I found I slept more soundly, my mind felt sharper, and I was enjoying feelings of simple anticipation and excitement.

On the morning the walk was scheduled to begin Mum and I sat in her kitchen eating porridge and listening to the ducks. I wasn't the slightest bit nervous or apprehensive, but there was a part of me that didn't want to leave – or rather didn't want to leave my mum. She had been my anchor, and the boat had been my sanctuary for two months, during the most tumultuous and confusing time of my life. I squeezed her so tightly as I got out of her car at the train station to go to Brighton, and felt a lump in my throat as she drove away. I was really going to miss her.

I hitched my pack on to the luggage rail and settled into the train seat. I watched the grey, stone streets of Essex rush by and within a couple of hours I arrived in Brighton. I wasn't keen on a big send-off. I just wanted to slip off quietly and start my adventure alone. My best friend, Freeman, however, was having none of that.

Freeman and I became friends in September 1997, on the school bus after the first day of secondary school. We spent the forty-minute journey back to Maldon on the front seats of the upper deck, falling boisterously into each other as the bus veered around corners and letting out high, prepubescent yelps whenever it hit bumps in the road. We couldn't believe there was no competition to get those seats and congratulated ourselves on discovering the funnest possible way to ride the bus home. (It was a week before we realized that the cool kids sat at the back.)

Freeman and I became inseparable and, twenty-three years since that bus ride, we remain a strong team. When I told him I was going to drop everything and walk around Britain, he honoured the occasion by clearing his schedule so as not to let his teammate begin a journey on his own.

Freeman hates Brighton, and although we spoke on the phone nearly every day in the years I lived there, he would only ever make the trip from his home in London if there was a good enough reason to. And so for him to come to the city he jokingly describes as 'full of dossers sitting about on the beach taking ketamine' told me he wasn't prepared to let me wander off into Britain's back country without his hand on my back. I definitely would have regretted not sharing that first day, my first steps on my 3,000(ish)-mile walk around Great Britain, with someone I love. That's why Freeman is my best mate: he knows what I need better than I do a lot of the time.

We sat for an hour or so on the benches outside the North Laine Brewhouse. Freeman looked very at home in a pair of jeans, a jumper and sunglasses, while I was testing out my new look – a blue base layer (hiking speak for 'a lightweight top'), my saucy new zip-off hiking trousers and my spanking-new walking boots. I wasn't entirely sure what Freeman made of this whole walking-around-Britain idea or how I'd arrived at the decision to do it. We'd spent our entire friendship smoking weed, listening to Tool and trying to make each other laugh. If anyone knows that I'm not an endurance athlete by nature, it's him. But as we sat there comfortably enjoying a pint, neither of us even spoke about what I was about to do. It was like it was just another thing that was happening; we knew we'd still be best mates once it was over, so what was the point in discussing it? Freeman told me a long time ago that I'm a bit of a mystery to him. That sometimes he simply doesn't understand me, or the things I do. The walk, I guess, was a good example of this: he didn't really get it, but he supported and encouraged me nonetheless. The fact that he was there was enough to show me he was proud of me, and although we didn't discuss how I was feeling about the walk or even how I was in myself particularly, him being there made me feel like he had my back, and that's all I needed.

Once we'd finished our drinks, we took a stroll down to the pier. The sun was peeking through more than predicted, making the colours of the grass and flower beds glow around the fountain at the Old Steine. I'm sure it would make great reading to say that I was nervous, excited, overwhelmed – all the emotions you might expect if you put yourself in my shoes – but in truth there was very little of that. The whole occasion was washing over me. I wasn't looking forwards or backwards – I was just there, experiencing it like it was any other day. When Freeman and I reached the pier, however, I felt a little surge of warmth, a tiny moment where everything inside and around me felt like it was all how it should be, and in that moment I could feel that the adventure was really happening. After a hug and a selfie, I faced west and began to walk.

I'd been down this road hundreds of times before. Kingsway, on Brighton's iconic seafront, is a stretch of sticky, seagull-shat asphalt that runs alongside the main road, overlooking the beach. As I slalomed through hordes of sunburnt day-trippers I felt like a ghost. I didn't belong in this crowd, not today. Brighton's gulls were in typically proud voice and provided the klaxon for the start of day one – a ten-mile toddle to the seaside town of Worthing. Despite having a brand-new tent at my disposal, I wasn't convinced that Worthing was the place to try it out. Conveniently, my friend Adam had been in touch a few days previously to ask when my walk was due to begin. After telling him my plan to walk to Worthing on the first day, he insisted I stay with him above The Bugle – a popular Worthing pub where he'd recently become the live-in general manager.

Usually, I'm not really one for planning. If anything, I take comfort in not knowing what my future looks like – which is probably why I was able to seriously consider a walk around Britain in the first place. But considering the scale of this undertaking, and the fact that it would become my life for the next seven months, I thought I should work out what I was going to do for the first week, when I was finding my feet. After Worthing, I plotted the places I planned to reach by the end of each day and made sure there would be somewhere I could camp. After the end of the first week I'd plot out the next week, and do the same week by week from there.

Kingsway became Albion Street as the tourist-trap of Brighton seafront turned into the industrial no-man's land that banks the River Adur. It was an unattractive start to the day, all told, and it wasn't until the copper lantern roof of Shoreham's iconic lighthouse, Kingston Buci, came into view that I felt like I was finally being treated to some of the maritime quaintness of East Sussex. Made from limestone collected from the Lewes Valley, Kingston Buci has kept a watchful eye over Shoreham harbour for over 150 years, and passing it felt like passing the first marker. In a 'Samwise Gamgee moment', I recognized that this was the furthest out of Brighton I had ever walked.

I rejoined the seafront after passing back across the Adur, and in doing so I was able to turn back and view the city in the middle distance. The first thing I noticed was the towering i360, a garish observation tower that is the all-time worst addition to Brighton seafront, an eyesore of eyesores, forever at odds with the landscape around it. In that moment it represented everything I hated about the life I was leaving behind.

After an hour or so meandering through residential streets to the sea I felt like I had to almost be in Worthing. I'd plotted what I thought to be a ten-mile walk, door to door from the Palace Pier to The Bugle, using the Ordnance Survey app – a legitimate mapping service that I'd agreed to pay a £5 monthly subscription for. Ten miles was plenty, I'd reasoned, for my first day of walking. It was a distance that, despite knowing it would be challenging, I was happy to complete. My pedometer had informed me that I had walked 9.2 miles from the pier, and over the past hour I'd been noticing a dull ache forming in my legs and a pain in my back that I'd been able to ignore. Seeing that I was just under a mile from completing my first day, I decided to switch to Google Maps so I could punch in the exact location of Adam's pub. It informed me I was – somehow – still 3.3 miles short of my final destination. The pain in my legs and back suddenly became so pronounced that I had to sit down and have a breather. It's amazing what a rush of disappointment can do to you physically. I took another look at my map.

How had this happened? How could it be ten miles on one app and twelve and a half on another?

I'd gone from feeling like Edward P. Weston (known as 'the greatest walker of all time' after walking from LA to New York in seventy-seven days) to Rab C. Nesbitt (a muttering, swearing oaf) in the blink of an eye. It wouldn't be the last time I would be let down by my navigation skills, or the last time I'd blame my apparatus for my own mistakes.

The last three miles hurt, and I'm embarrassed to admit that. I'd swanned into this thing assuming I'd be able to just do it, with no real training and no real plan. An hour later I hobbled on to Marine Parade with all the form of a ninety-year-old. I'd arrived in Worthing at around 6 p.m., five hours after I'd left Brighton, exhausted, embarrassed and well and truly spent.

Half an hour later, I reached the pub. It sounded busy and

I had a hunch that attempting to shove myself and my enormous pack through the bar would result in me having to replace several spilt pints. I sent Adam a message asking him to meet me out the back, where, to my relief, there was an entirely unoccupied beer garden. I hobbled through the gate, unclipped the straps of my pack and let it crash to the ground. The idea of carrying it around the country suddenly felt deeply demoralizing. My thighs were screaming, my back, too; I felt like I'd just carried a dead cow up several flights of stairs. The soles of my feet were sore, and I wondered how much worse it would have been if I'd walked to Worthing across the shingle beach barefoot. Not much.

For the first of what was to be many times, worry crept in. Consumed by my vision of the perfect adventure and drunk on the applause of my friends and family, it was clear I'd developed a somewhat cavalier attitude towards how big a challenge this was going to be. My physical pain was replaced by something far more uncomfortable – anxiety filled my blood and crept over my skin – as I realized that I'd *hugely* underestimated the walk.

A moment later I heard Adam's voice as he approached the back door. I tried to get up and the pain jabbed my thighs once more. God I felt wrecked.

The door swung open and Adam, clutching a half-drunk pint of lager, stepped out and took in the state of me. He didn't need to ask how my day had been, he just held his glass aloft and said with a mischievous smile, 'Come on, mate, my round.'

Warmth washed over me. *Alcohol.* All my anxieties, my dread and, if I was lucky, my aches and pains, would soon be washed away. Good old Ads. Good old booze.

The pub was bigger than I expected, and was nice, I guess. It had all the hallmarks of a traditional pub that had been recently renovated, but a decent boozer, I decided.

I left my pack at the back door and limped towards the bar. A throng of regulars was assembled there, at first glance a typically salt-of-the-earth bunch, awkward and comfortable in equal measure, as men of a certain age tend to be when they gather in the pub – all belly laughs and pensive sips. They'd formed a tight wall of polo shirts, faded forearm tattoos and beer guts and for a moment I was riled at the thought of having to fight my way through to be served, but as soon as Adam got back behind the bar he introduced me and told them my story (he referred to it as a 'sponsored walk', much to my annoyance; *this isn't exactly the annual Maldon sponsored walk and barbecue, Ads*), and then they refused to let me pay for my drinks. Or ask for them. The evening turned out to be a constant battle between me trying to finish my beer and having the next one put in front of me. Freeman, who had wisely opted for a twenty-minute train ride to get to Worthing over a six-hour walk, had arrived an hour or so after I did, bringing with him a clutch of tagalongs who had decided to celebrate the end of the first day with me. Today *was* a celebration – or that's how I justified it to myself – so I knocked back each drink that was put in front of me, accordingly.

It wasn't long before I was tremendously pissed and I had indeed forgotten all the uneasy feelings I'd had in the garden, all my aches and pains and, it would seem, the walk itself.

At this stage in my life, I'd got into the habit of counteracting my self-critical thoughts and the feeling that I have no genuine relationships either by surrounding myself with big personalities (confident, outspoken, self-assured people whose ability to interact without fear of being judged sometimes allows me to feel the same) or by getting drunk. As I'm sure is the case with many people, my ability to function

39

socially is greatly enhanced after I get four beers and two shots in me. However (and I'm probably not revealing anything new here), this isn't exactly a sustainable model for happiness. In fact, I'd say that for every occasion I've reached for a drink to help loosen me up, I've had to pay for it with anything between two and seven days of misery, nervousness, paranoia and regret. So why do I always go back to it?

It had been a long time since my first bar shift at Malone's Diner, a family-run American restaurant at the top end of Maldon High Street. I fell in love with the job, but also became excited by the person it allowed me to become. I liked the whole 'barman' shtick, the theatre of bartending; I loved that I was the person responsible for loosening everyone up, for helping folks take a load off and just enjoy themselves. It did for them what I wanted for me, so I began doing what they did. Drinking. Not just to have a good time, but to have just one evening where I could, in effect, get away from myself.

It wasn't long before I realized just how much better I was at working behind the bar after a couple of shots. I was able to up my game – make people laugh, get into interesting conversations, earn more tips . . . And now I'd discovered what booze could do, it quickly bled into my social life, as I suppose it does for most eighteen-year-olds. Being drunk was essentially a shortcut to becoming the version of Jake I like; it helped me accept who I was – something I was so desperate for – and, what's more, I felt it turned me into the type of person that people wanted to be around. But, as we all know, what goes up must come down, and despite being young enough for hangovers not to be the near-death experience they are these days, the day after a hefty binge was always savage, not so much in a sicky, headachey way, more in a sad, lonely and befuddled way – the type of hangover that can't be shifted with two Nurofen, a bottle of Lucozade and two packets of Space Raiders. This continued throughout my twenties, and as the years went on and the drinking got heavier, and more regular, depression became routine . . . and that's before I even *mention* recreational drugs.

I discovered cocaine when I first moved to Brighton in the summer of 2007. I'd taken hard drugs sporadically before – ecstasy, mushrooms and a little speed during my late teens, and had, to be honest, had a great time experimenting. The times I spent sitting in a field or a mate's garden completely cabbaged, talking passionately about how wonderful the world would be if everyone took mushrooms, I truly believe turned me into a more open-minded and thoughtful individual. Coke, however, is a nonsense drug that should never be taken by anybody. I started taking it occasionally at first, and loved the refreshing burst of confident energy it gave me, but it didn't take me long to realize that that feeling usually lasts about five minutes and the rest of the evening is spent chasing that initial high. Where shrooms and alcohol provided me with a temporary gateway to the version of me I like, cocaine kicked down a door in some disgusting recessed back alley of my mind where all the blinds are drawn and there are anxious little versions of me running around shouting at each other. It turns everyone who takes it into the least fun, least relaxed, most annoying version of themselves, and it's somehow managed to convince huge swathes of British drinkers that no night is complete without it.

My mental-health troubles definitely became more severe when I started involving coke in every drinking session. My thoughts became dark and tangled, more and more with each line. There's something indefinably sinister and underhand about coke; not only did it tend to reverse the good feeling I set out to accomplish by getting drunk, it often replaced it with a shady, ominous anxiety that was impossible to shake off. And yet, because of its sheer chemical addictiveness, there's *still* always a part of the night where I start thinking about it, and the process of thinking about it generally impedes any sort of enjoyment until the moment my house key appears under my nostril . . . which is, I'm afraid to write, precisely what happened on the first night, at the end of the first day of my walk around Britain.

Needless to say, I feel the appropriate amount of guilt for allowing that first night to get as out of hand as it did. I could have left my recklessness out of this story, and got away with it. But, because it's a near-faultless example of the way my destructive cycle works, it's kind of pivotal to the whole thing. I felt anxious to the point of overwhelmed in Adam's beer garden, so I took something (alcohol) to counteract it and, as ever, it worked its charm. Once the glow of being drunk had worn off, doing a 'cheeky line' I was offered perked me right up. I spent the next six hours chasing the good feeling I got at the start of the night with more booze, and more drugs, but with every sip and every line I just went down further until all I was was a need for nothing more than wanting more. By the time the sun came up I was a horrendous cocktail of regret, paranoia, blocked nostrils and nervous exhaustion . . . and I still had sleep to contend with.

Adam showed me to the spare room on the first floor. Daylight poured through the curtainless windows, he pointed to a lifeless beige futon in the corner, reminded me what a 'top night' we'd had and closed the door.

I woke up with a cough and a splutter a few hours later. It was 1 p.m. I felt horrible. But I *had* to make a move. I *had* to.

When I got downstairs into the bar Ads was nowhere to

be seen. I poked my half-blocked nose around in a vague attempt to spot him then, with a deep, dejected breath, strode with mock purpose towards the front door and weakly pushed it open. A gust of cold, wet wind slapped me across the face as I peered out in the direction I'd planned to walk.

Day two was ten miles again, this time inland, into the chalk hills of the South Downs, to Arundel. I'd meet my brother in the town. Sam had decided a few days previously to get a train down from London and spend day three walking across the downs with me to Chichester, fifteen or so miles east of Arundel. I'd been really excited about seeing him, but now, staring blankly down the road through bloodshot eyes, waiting half-heartedly for something, anything, that might get me out of taking those first steps, all I wanted to do was crawl under something soft and never speak to anyone ever again. For a second I imagined the comfort of the duvet I'd spent a month under on Mum's boat.

I groaned, sloped out of the pub and trudged pathetically up the road, clenching my jaw.

Destructive behaviour is a big and complicated part of depression. Over the course of many years and many low times, I've managed to sabotage myself in many ways – drinking, taking drugs, breaking things, arguing, cancelling plans, eating too much, not eating at all, missing deadlines, not talking, not brushing my teeth, not tidying my house, staying up too late, not getting out of bed, not moving, putting things off, disregarding consequences, over-sharing, isolating, seeking validation through sex, avoiding loved ones, maintaining toxic relationships . . . you get the idea.

Sometimes I'll wilfully enter into damaging behaviours, knowing that it's likely to tip me over the edge. Maybe it's to feel like I have some control. Or maybe it's because I feel like, if I'm hurting myself directly, then there's no room for anyone, or anything, else to hurt me. I can't be let down further if I'm already at the bottom. I win . . . in a way.

It makes sense that vices are what we turn to when we're feeling low. They provide pleasure, if only temporary. I know from experience that cocooning myself in a duvet, ignoring my friends and smoking weed all day is, on balance, significantly less exhausting than putting on a mask and pretending life's fine when it isn't. That's why it's important to remember that while indulging in the 'comfort of being sad' by not getting out of bed, or getting off your face, or ignoring messages from friends might feel like it's absolutely what you need, it's also worth being mindful of small things you can do to balance the scales a bit. I know what it's like when you're so depressed that even the thought of stepping out of your front door is enough to make you want to vomit. But there are other things, equally constructive, you can do that aren't quite so alarming. Make your bed, cook yourself something simple, put a clothes wash on, respond to one email, brush your hair, open your window, breathe in some fresh air . . . To someone buckling under the weight of depression, it's important to see these tasks as victories, proof that you are a capable, functioning human being. Big or small, if a task feels constructive, then it is, and if it required effort to do it, then you deserve praise for doing it. People who run a marathon in under three hours might be the most proficient, but what about the runners who finish in seven hours? They're out there on the course way longer, digging in way beyond what's comfortable, unrelenting to the point of collapse. In some ways they deserve more praise than the winner.

For me, the damaging behaviours had gone on too long, and I had given myself no praise for my 'little victories'. In the end, I had to be honest with myself about whether going easy on myself for ignoring my friends or congratulating myself six days in a row for just taking a shower was really encouraging a shift towards getting better. What I needed was a little self-discipline. I had to take charge. I needed to force myself to do some things I didn't want to, or couldn't be arsed to, in order to start feeling better (like walking Reggie). Balancing on the line between constructive criticism and liberal praise is really difficult, but knowing that's what you have to do is a really good start to feeling more confident in yourself.

That dreary afternoon, after a moment of mournful trudging and contemplating whether I was really about to attempt to walk ten miles, mostly uphill, in the pissing rain, when I felt this glum, I stopped in my tracks and thought about what the sensible move was. *If I go back to Ad's, I reckon I could sleep for a good fifteen hours and still get up and out the door early enough tomorrow morning to walk to Arundel and meet Sam.* It was a six-out-of-ten plan, far from ideal, but it would do.

5

My alarm went off at 6 a.m. I had, remarkably, managed to sleep for fifteen hours, as planned. I actually felt good – rested and eager to pack up my things and go to meet my brother. There's something about starting a day early that really energizes me these days. In all the years I worked in bars I was always jealous when I overheard the quiet, unperturbed sounds of 'morning people' – housemates pottering around the kitchen making tea and toast and listening to Radio 6 at a diplomatic volume. I would often start and finish work at such antisocial hours that it was extremely rare for anybody to catch a glimpse of me before midday, so waking up early now feels like I've created time out of thin air.

Worthing was still fast asleep. My legs and back had recovered and as I began to head north into the crisp morning air I was filled with a renewed sense of purpose. I'd made mistakes on the first day, but that was all behind me now. I was bound to make a few in the early stages – I'm still me, after all.

The best route into the South Downs was via the village of Findon, a modest three-mile trot north from The Bugle. From there I would head west towards Arundel via a section of what appeared to be one of Britain's longest and most aimless footpaths – the Monarch's Way. It acts as a sort of tribute to King Charles II's clandestine escape to Europe after having his royal arse handed to him at the Battle of Worcester. I couldn't help but think that, with the non-stop development of southern England since the Civil War, the path is probably about as true to Charles's route to exile as Mel Gibson's depiction in *Braveheart* is to the real William Wallace. That said, there's history there, and as I followed the Monarch's Way through the chalk hills of the South Downs I enjoyed thinking about the historical significance of where I was – something I couldn't remember ever doing before.

I continued west, taking in everything around me: the damp of the morning that made the country smell more like itself; the sound of the trees as the breeze ushered me through the long, winding bridleways of Wepham Wood. The sky overhead was grey, but the colour of the woods around me was as vibrant as it could possibly be. I'd walked far enough now that there was no visible sign of civilization, and as I stood alone, breathing deep lungfuls of unsullied air among the deciduous trees and fallen leaves all around me, I felt grateful. Like it had all been put there that morning, just for me.

There's something about nature that is so undeniably good for our mental health. For me, it's a reminder that this world was here billions of years before me and will (hopefully) be here billions of years after I'm gone. Something about that really helps put my problems into perspective. Seeing the sun rise or set, watching the tide coming in and out, it makes the world feel magical, and it makes you feel special, like you've somehow ended up in a perfect place at a perfect time. But it happens every single day, everywhere, even if you don't see it.

I arrived in Arundel just after midday and, despite a general 'long-walk' feeling in my legs, I was free from any real pain and felt like I still had plenty of gas left in the tank.

Arundel is stunning – a market town seeped in quaint English charm, with a crooked high street lined with inns and shops held together by sturdy black beams selling local produce.

I took my map out – a crisp, new Ordnance Survey map of the Arundel and Pulborough area my friend Phil had bought for me as a gift. I had planned on using my OS maps app for the duration of the walk, but Phil, a man very hot on things being done correctly, insisted it was a matter of absolute necessity that I learn how to read a map properly. He invited me over to his place one night and presented me with a bundle of OS maps and a baseplate compass, an instrument that until then I had no idea existed. He spent a good hour teaching me how to use it – an hour that, as I sat dimly fumbling with it at Arundel station while I waited for my brother, turned out had been completely wasted on me. I gave up on the compass but studied the map until I was sure enough that I knew where we were heading. I'd suggested to Sam that we still attempt to walk the thirteen miles to Chichester, a plan that now seemed ambitious, considering the time we'd end up setting off.

As my brother's train pulled up I put my map back in its plastic sheath (sexy) and hung it around my neck. I knew my new hiking look would amuse him so I thought I'd milk it a bit, despite the fact that it hadn't exactly been plain sailing the past couple of days and I was miles away from becoming the seasoned hiker I was making myself out to be.

As he walked towards me I saw him looking me up and down.

'Hey, man,' I said.

'Hey.' He smirked. 'You look like a poster boy for Millets.'

I always feel a bit like the 'first pancake' whenever I hang out with my younger brother, like my parents fluffed their first attempt and after adjusting the mix and getting the heat right the next one came out much better-looking, much cleverer, more quick-witted and better in social situations than the first one. I wouldn't say I've ever really been jealous of

48

Sam, but I've always admired him – he's a brilliant person and I'm proud that he's my brother.

Sam was hosting a weekly show on London Fields radio at the time and had told me a week or so previously that he was keen to join me at different sections of my walk to record our conversations in the hope of turning it into 'something'. I loved the idea. I felt that listening to a recording of me and my brother in years to come would transport me back to that time way better than any photo.

After successfully negotiating us out of town I checked the map again when we reached what I assumed was the way into Arundel Park. I worked out that if I could guide us through the park and on to the South Downs Way we'd be able to follow the trail most of the way to Chichester. Once we were in the park, surrounded by nature, despite the drizzle I felt that inner peace again. The grass glowed brilliant green all about, wrapping itself around every inch of the hills as perfectly as felt on a snooker table. Once again there was no civilization, no one else, and for a brief moment in that valley I felt like my brother and I were the only people on Earth.

Sam decided, quite rightly, that this was an ideal moment to get something on tape and liberated his recording device from his bag. After some good-quality froth while he got the sound levels right he tried to get some context out of me by asking about my reasons for doing the walk – and I became suddenly aware that I hadn't ever spoken to him about what had been going on with me.

Speaking openly about depression was still a relatively new thing for me at this point. I still hadn't fully formed my thoughts on what it all meant, exactly, or what had happened to me in east London. I hadn't considered the possibility that I might have to get into it with those closest to me, to make the details of a traumatic experience palatable for my loved ones. I'd spoken to my mum and a doctor at the very peak of my meltdown, and then to Irene, the CBT therapist, but I hadn't spoken about it in any depth since that time.

Entering into a discussion with my brother about my mental health felt precarious. I was afraid that communicating how close I'd been to taking my own life would needlessly shake the foundations of our strong relationship. We'd never been down this road before and it was impossible to tell how it would sit with him. I felt protective; I didn't want to divide my pain up and give him half of it, like it was the last Bourbon in Nan's biscuit barrel.

Sam's always been someone who doesn't feel the need to weigh into a topic if he doesn't have to. He's an exceptionally good listener and always encourages me to talk until I come to whatever point it is I'm trying to make. Thankfully, that day I was on a pretty even keel and able to speak freely about my mental health without being too explicit about how painful the past year had been for me and, despite being anxious about it at first, I felt our relationship strengthen as we talked.

Something about speaking to him about it for his podcast made the process a little easier, too, a little less like a confessional, and as we could turn off the device whenever we wanted to, it felt like we didn't have to talk about it and nothing else.

Sam and I can chat away happily for hours, but our conversations are typically more about the nature of humans in general, or music or football. This level of soul-baring was a little above our usual station, and the thing I noticed was that the more we talked, the more I understood that this wasn't going to be a discussion that had an end point. The subject matter obviously carried a ton of extra weight, but it seemed the main encumbrance wasn't actually having the talk itself but starting it – in the same way that getting yourself out of the front door is often the most difficult part of going for a run. I suppose the trick to ensuring you don't have to re-open the conversation is to keep the door on the latch. It's a heavy door and it takes a great deal of strength to open it. It's just not practical, then, to let it fall closed after just one chat.

The weight of the conversation is often the barrier that stops people opening up to each other, and I believe it's because we all worry that by sharing our problems we're going to put some of that weight on to someone else's shoulders. But telling someone that you have a problem doesn't mean that they then have it. Sure, it's not going to be pleasant for them to hear, but that's only because they love you, and because they're worried about you. *You're* the one in pain. Sharing it won't hurt them the way it's hurting you. Give the people who actually give a shit about you a chance to do what they're there for. To love and support you and help you through when life gets hard. That's the bottom line of what friends are. You can be acquaintances with anyone. Your loved ones are the people you're *supposed* to go through things with. You are part of their world, and they desperately want you to be.

The drizzle had turned to rain and Arundel Park grew increasingly muddy so our conversation meandered away from feelings and on to the terrain. After one or two near-calamitous slips we reached a fortified structure that seemed to be another entrance to the park from a main road on the other side. We hadn't expected that. We'd been walking for a couple of hours by this point, and there had definitely been more than a little guesswork on my part with regard to which direction we should be heading in. We stopped and took a closer look at the map.

I pointed to a main road that, unbeknownst to us, had been running parallel to the valley the entire time. We were now at a place called 'Whiteway's Lodge', next to a big roundabout that connects the A284 and the A29. Shit.

'We're out of our depth, aren't we?' Sam said. 'On day one of map-reading.'

I looked down at my OS map; previously crisp, it now sat uselessly in my hands, sodden and crumbling away in the rain.

The slim chance of us making it to Chichester was now gone so, not through want or lack of endeavour, Sam and I reluctantly agreed that the only option left was to turn around and head back to Arundel.

The return journey seemed to take half the time, and there was even time to cheer our effort along over a warming dram of whisky in a local pub before Sam's train arrived. We were weary, but not dispirited; in fact, despite my failings at orienteering, I was in high spirits from spending such a heartfelt and calamitous afternoon with my brother. As I waved him off I felt a surge of determination and decided that, rather than fully admitting defeat and spending my first night wild camping on this walk on the outskirts of town, I'd attempt to navigate my way back into the South Downs, properly this time, and set up camp somewhere away from civilization. No more showing off by vaguely referring to the map at random points, no rattling off stock terms like 'contour line' to impress my brother, and no claiming to know exactly where I was at all times. It was just me now, and I was going to take it seriously this time.

Back in Arundel Park, I followed the correct trail up a sharp bank. The grass was sodden and as I tried to grind in one heavy boot in front of the other for grip, my legs suddenly processed the hours I'd been on my feet that day and sent waves of lava down my thighs and into my calves. The exertion of our afternoon had made me forget all about the half-marathon I'd walked from Worthing, but now my body was remembering every step. For the first time that day I began to resent walking, and with each demanding lunge the burn got deeper and my desire to stop and sit down supplanted my determination to get out of Arundel. Once again, the reality of circumnavigating the British mainland wasn't in keeping with the serene, Tolkienesque vision I'd had of it before setting off, and as I dragged myself despairingly to the top of the embankment, my feeling towards walking three thousand miles in seven months switched from 'moderately challenging' to 'fucking absurd'.

Looking back now, I wonder what difference it would have made to those first few days if I'd forced myself to be a bit more pragmatic, to visualize the true scale and seriousness of my challenge. It might have removed the temptation to get off my face in Worthing on the first night, and maybe if I'd spent some time developing essential skills I wouldn't have cost myself an afternoon by casting Sam and me wildly adrift on the outskirts of Arundel. I'd been so preoccupied by the mental-health side of the walk I'd overlooked some vital practical steps.

It took several wheezing minutes to scale the bank. It plateaued and I felt a moment of relief as a cool breeze whipped through my hair. I felt drained but ignored the urge to crouch, not trusting myself enough to get back up again if I did. I steeled myself and began shuffling, wearily, through a flattened trail that ran through long, windswept grass. A cold air current swarmed across the higher ground, dancing through the grass and shaking my damp clothes away from my skin. I checked the map once more to make certain I was on the right path and plodded in the direction of Houghton. I'd clocked up almost twenty miles, and I was feeling it, but the thought of having to play catch-up again the following day was just too dispiriting and so, with a little self-compassion, I urged myself forward, maintaining a gentle pace for another half an hour or so. I came to a turn-off leading me up a very steep flight of steps, and that took me straight on to the South Downs Way. A few wincing minutes of pins and needles, then onwards, following the trail for a couple of miles to Eartham Wood. It appeared that my body was capable of far more than I gave it credit for, and I felt something almost resembling triumph, a comfortable confidence in how I'd fared, a belief that I might actually be able to do this after all.

By eight o'clock, however, dusk had settled in, and after that brief wave of pride had evaporated the prospect of spending a night alone in a tent was beginning to make me nervous. I found a small clearing and, with the light nearly gone and no other options in sight, it seemed a suitable enough spot. While I may have been a little cavalier in much of my approach to this walk, when it came to choosing a tent I'm pleased to say I'd done my homework. Hours spent trawling through various outdoor-goods websites, camping forums and insufferable YouTube reviews (they all began, it seemed, with the same thirty-eight-year-old virgin in a yellow gilet kneeling earnestly beside a perfectly erected tent and addressing the viewers as 'guys') had resulted in what felt like just the thing to call home during a walk around Britain – the Wild Country Zephyros 2.

Keen to distance myself from the type of 'outdoorsman' I saw in those videos – the kind who refers to products by their full name – I decided to name my tent 'the Flea', a nod to 'The Zephyr Song' by Red Hot Chili Peppers. It was a name that would become more and more appropriate as the weeks went on and 'the Flea' became more and more revolting.

Although that night on the downs was to be the Flea's maiden overnight voyage, it had been out of its sheath once, while I was out walking Reggie at the Maldon Prom the previous month. I'd taken it out so I could spend a good twenty minutes making sure all the pieces were there and there were no holes in it, and to learn how to put it up. This level of meticulousness was new for me, and a far cry from the complete lack of respect I used to show my tents in my festival-going days – every erection being either a botched attempt following several warm pints of Carling or a complete rush job after arriving late and in a mad dash to the Concrete Jungle to catch The Mars Volta.

My prep work paid off. It took only a few minutes to slot every pole, peg and guy rope into place and I was ready to cross the threshold and make myself at home. I crawled in, leaving my feet outside, and smiled as I heard the first plinks of rain bounce off the roof. I slowly removed my walking boots. You know when people ask what you'd do if you had three wishes? Well, before eternal life, a billion quid, world peace, all of that, I think I'd choose to live in a perpetual sensation of feeling like I'm slowly taking my boots off. After walking twenty miles in a day it's honestly the single greatest sensation I've ever experienced.

I shuffled into my new sleeping bag and laid back, stretching my arms behind my head and exhaling as loudly as I've ever exhaled. What a bloody day.

The following morning, after a nervy first night where every little crack and snuffle outside my tent sounded like something enormous that might kill me, I kicked myself out of my sleeping bag and unzipped my front door so that I could get a better sense of where I was.

The landscape that had felt so close and oppressive in the dark was now wide open and the air was warm with promising notes of summer. The untidy melodies of hundreds of birds whistled playfully all around me. Within the few moments I spent silently gazing across the countryside the fear from the night disappeared, washed away like a sketch in the sand. And so began a morning routine that would span the length of my tour of Britain. Starting each day in silent appreciation of the natural world allowed me not just to recentre but to achieve focus in a way that only being in nature can. As I packed the rest of my things up, disassembled the Flea and stuffed everything back into my pack I realized that despite my bumpy sleep I couldn't wait to get going. I took a quick look at the map to make sure I was heading in the right direction then hoisted my pack on to my shoulders and continued along the trail, leaving nothing in my wake but a small area of dry, slightly flattened grass.

I really believe that one of the most life-affirming things a human can do is spend a few days hiking. The process of walking for miles surrounded by trees and fields, finding a place to camp, spending the night in the wild and packing everything away again the following morning and continuing to walk is as close as most of us can get to testing what we were designed for. I interviewed the author Matt Haig once, who said, 'Human beings are essentially 30,000-year-old hardware trying to run twenty-first-century software. It's no wonder we crash now and again.' That's how I felt that morning – like I was doing what I was designed to do.

I spent the next few days with my head down, moseying through beautiful West Sussex and Hampshire villages. I felt a sense of urgency that had so far eluded me, and headed west as straight and as quickly as the crow flies to make up the time I'd lost in the first few days. I squelched from one side of the small sailing village of Bosham, four miles west of Chichester, to the other across the bay, through wet seaweed and among hundreds of marooned boats and happy dogs chasing each other.

I was stopped on the way to Havant on the West Sussex/ Hampshire border, a further five miles west, by a man in a much-worn pair of hiking boots who called out to me to enquire about my rucksack. His name was Neil, and he was a seasoned hiker with the calm soul and weathered skin to back it up. He wore a plain black T-shirt that hung off him like he'd been wearing it every day for a year, and when he asked me how far I planned on walking his grey eyes sparkled and widened enough that the crow's feet around his eyes momentarily disappeared. Apart from the old boys at Adam's pub (which didn't really count, because they were absolutely steaming), it was the first proper reaction to my walk I'd experienced, and after I'd told him my route and why I was doing it, he told me not just how he'd covered a lot of the ground in Scotland that I was planning to – the West Highland Way, the Great Glen Way, the Cairngorms – but also that he had recently lost his mum and was getting back into walking as a way to get his head together. I didn't know it at the time, but that chat with Neil provided me with a blueprint I'd use again and again in the hundreds of surprisingly open, honest conversations I'd have with strangers over the following months. It was a pleasure to chat to someone who, in that moment at least, felt something like a kindred spirit – a person hurt and with a mountain to climb, but willing to dig in and just get on with it.

I continued west into Hampshire, along the Ports Down ridge that overlooks Portsmouth Harbour. In the far distance I could just make out the Spinnaker Tower, which, although it spoilt the view for me a little, is a far more tasteful addition to Portsmouth's coastline than the i360 is to Brighton's. Somewhere between Southampton and Fareham, after another few nervy nights in the tent, I decided to fork out for a patch of grass on a campsite, just so I could get a solid night's sleep free of anxiety about sudden violent death.

I was about twenty minutes from reaching the campsite when it started to rain. I upped my pace in a fairly futile attempt to get there quicker, but then a car pulled up alongside me. The driver's-side window came down to reveal an elderly woman, looking very concerned.

'Goodness me, where are you heading?' she asked. Her hair was thin and white like a cloud and her hands looked so soft and delicate as they perched at 10-2 on her steering wheel.

'Oh, just up here,' I replied. 'There's a campsite at the next turn-off.'

'Let me run you over there. You're soaked!'

She wasn't wrong, it was really pissing it down and, considering the campsite really was only a couple of minutes away, I decided that taking her up on her charitable offer probably wouldn't quite constitute cheating. I jumped in the passenger side after bundling my pack into the back and off we went at a leisurely 15 mph towards my home for the evening. I told her what I was doing – I'd never really summed up my entire vision for the walk and how I'd come to do it before – and when she pulled into the campsite and stopped the car it was clear she didn't know what to make of it at all. After a few moments she said: 'Do you have plans for dinner?'

I was a bit taken aback. I'd never received an invitation like that from a stranger and, despite there being nothing immediately intimidating about her, or her invitation, the fact that it had happened at all was enough to put me slightly on edge. Why would someone invite a drifter over to their house for no reason?

I didn't want to say either yes or no so I asked if she'd mind coming back in an hour after I'd set my tent up. It felt like a genuine offer, an incredibly kind and neighbourly one, but I couldn't shake the sense of danger I felt. *There must be a reason she's invited me round. What is it? Has she done this before? Did she say 'family', or am I making that up? What if it's like the Manson family? What if she has two sons at hers, sharpening knives and putting on gimp masks right now?*

I didn't want to miss an opportunity to spend a serendip-itous evening with a very, very kind person, but neither did I want to end up being turned into 'art' and mounted above a mad old lady's mantelpiece. I decided that I *would* go with her when she came back, but that I would do these four things to cover my back just in case it did end up turning into a real life Rob Zombie movie:

1. Take a photo of her number plate.
2. Open 'maps' on my phone and take a screenshot when we arrive at her house.
3. Send both photos to Mum.
4. Tell Mum to call me an hour after I'd been picked up; then, if I was getting bad vibes I could pretend the call was from the campsite, telling me my tent had been ransacked and I had to go back immediately.

I thought these four steps would be enough to provide me with a sense of safety until I arrived at the woman's house and deemed it all clear ... which, of course, it was. After picking me up and driving us five minutes down the road, my host pulled into her driveway, where I was greeted cheer-fully by her very friendly-looking husband and equally friendly-looking daughter. They were the Brown family – Elaine, Gwyn, Philippa and Wellington the dog – and damn did they know how to make a guy feel welcome: olives and red wine out on the table, a tour of the house and garden and an introduction to their chickens, followed by a rustic, per-fectly cooked chicken dinner. When I received the call from Mum an hour later I was so engrossed in a slightly tipsy conversation with Gwyn I'd completely forgotten about my contingency plan. I answered the phone and felt so bad for putting such measures in place against sweet old completely harmless Elaine that I very swiftly got off the phone to Mum, went back through to the kitchen, ate another olive and told the Browns exactly what the point of the phone call was, much to their amusement.

As with most people, I'm sure, I've grown up with the assumption that if an offer seems too good to be true, it probably is. People often expect something in return for a good deed, and there's this idea that, at their core, everyone is only really looking out for themselves. So when I was met by Elaine's generosity, my instinct, sadly, was to treat it with the level of suspicion that should probably be reserved for politicians, cold callers and letting agents. Once we'd finished dinner and the last of the wine Elaine drove me back to the campsite. As I lay in my tent all warm and boozy and full of chicken, I listened to the rain and thought about that evening. I couldn't remember ever having felt so grateful, so gobsmacked by someone's generosity. Whether Elaine had shown her best, most caring side by inviting me in that evening, or if that's just how she was, her kindness was something that deserved to be acknowledged. It had only been six days since I left Brighton, and already the world had opened up.

6

Although Brighton was where I began my career in hospitality, I originally moved to the coast to fulfil my dream of becoming a musician. I'd wanted to be in a band ever since coming home from school in Year 6 and finding my dad sitting by the stereo in our old living room, hunched over his Washburn semi-acoustic guitar and trying to work out the chords to a track off the new Oasis record. When he saw me watching him, Dad paused the CD, handed over his guitar and patiently positioned my sticky child fingers into an E major shape. From that first strum I was hooked, and within a few months I'd taught myself a few more chords and started a 'band' with my best friend and a new kid in our class. A month before the summer holidays we convinced our headmaster to let us play at the end-of-year assembly. We were shocking. All we had was one microphone, one acoustic guitar and one electric guitar. I still remember so clearly looking across the assembly hall to see my then girlfriend (whatever that means in Year 6) sitting right at the back, head crumpled in her lap, hands clasped on the back of her head. It bordered on traumatic. My confidence was shot, and it remained shot for years.

I fell in love with music and spent my teens going to lots of gigs, but I was always too nervous to start my own band. But I stuck at my instrument, and by the time I moved to Brighton in 2007 enough time had passed for me to feel confident enough to give the band thing another shot. I initially convinced my friend Dan, who'd also moved to Brighton from Maldon, to start a band with me. Several years and many average songs later, Dan and his wife, Nic, moved to Southampton. Seven days and eighty miles after leaving Brighton's Palace Pier in 2016, I again found myself convincing Dan to help me out, this time asking him for a place to stay.

Dan and I didn't properly meet until I was about nineteen. I knew who he was before we became friends, but only as 'that mental bass player in that pop punk band'. While I dread to think of what's happened to the local music scene in Essex since rock music was all but wiped away from the British mainstream, back then there was still a real appetite for heavy music, which resulted in lots of decent local bands and an exciting live-music scene. Dan's band, Cousin Joey, were legends on the Essex circuit, renowned for high-octane performances and their ludicrously uplifting pop-punk cover of Katrina and the Waves' classic 'Walking on Sunshine'. Among the big personalities that made up that band, I always found Dan to be the most mesmerizing on stage, and I wasn't the only one; if they were on the bill, a Cousin Joey set was always the highlight of the night, and Dan would always be the highlight of the performance, tearing around the stage like a kid after too much orange squash.

Back then Dan was a local legend – a jolly, chunky, quiffed punk rocker who wore turned-up jeans, drank Maldon Gold and was the centre of attention in whatever pub he was in. When he wasn't charming the pants off everyone he met, he worked in the video-rental shop he owned, Videomania, and it was through a mutual love of horror movies that we eventually became friends. He's one of the best people I know, and I was so excited to be staying with him.

I arrived at Dan and Nic's place late in the afternoon, after a particularly uninspiring 12-mile yomp along the A roads from Fareham. I hadn't seen Dan properly in over a year and when he opened his front door and I saw that beaming smile of his I pounced on him with all the love I had to give. He looked great – his teenage puppy fat had become a thing of the past a couple of years previously when he decided to take up boxing, and he was now lean and sporting a newly shaved head and a big, thick beard.

Once we got settled, the three of us ate dinner, drank wine and talked about old times. It was ace. I got to chat to them a little more about my reasons for doing the walk, how happy it was making me to feel free after feeling so manacled and miserable in London. It was interesting to talk to Dan about emotions; it wasn't a topic we'd opened up as friends before. As with most of my close friendships, our history revolves around trying to make each other laugh. While he's a deeply kind person, and I probably always knew I could confide in him, I never did, because what really seemed to make me feel better if I ever felt down or anxious or not quite myself back then was the arsing around, the good-natured piss-taking, the not taking myself (or anything, for that matter) too seriously.

While I do of course advocate for establishing open, honest dialogue about mental health with loved ones, for me there's always been a time and a place for trying to forget about it all too. Sometimes I resist the urge to talk about how I'm feeling because I don't like the idea of amplified sympathy. While the empathy that comes from a response like 'It's OK, you're being so brave' works for me in the right moment, it can sometimes make me feel a bit pathetic, which *really* doesn't help. If I know someone well enough, sometimes a change of tack is appreciated. If a friend or family member notices I'm a bit off and I don't seem to want to talk about it, saying something funny or even taking the piss slightly often makes me laugh, and that allows me to cross the bridge between 'I'm fine' and 'Actually, I'm struggling a bit at the moment.'

Pushing emotions down, glossing over the hurt because the thought of revealing it is often followed by the fear of being labelled a downer – the balancing act of wallowing in private while pissing around in public felt like an effective enough approach for me back in the day. Although there's still a time and a place for it now, as I got older it felt like the good times and the laughs weren't quite enough to weather the more severe storms, so rather than fall into familiar social habits with Dan I felt like it was important to try what was for me at this point the *new* way. Speaking to Dan openly that night about how I'd been feeling the last few months and years was surprisingly easy; it didn't get as deep as it could – we still mostly wanted to have a laugh and catch up – but we spoke about feelings enough to connect on a couple of things, and that felt really good. I feel like it strengthened our friendship even.

'You said you feel in the moment now,' said Dan, taking a sip of his wine, planting his glass carefully on the table and leaning back into the sofa.

'Yeah,' I said. 'Like not worrying about the past or being anxious about the future, just being where I am and experiencing what's around me.'

'Hm,' said Dan quizzically. 'I feel like that's what I'm doing all the time, though.'

The fact that this was Dan's reality was news to me. I thought living in the moment was something everyone craved but always found difficult to achieve. I mean, it made sense, Dan being the type of person he is, but still I found the idea of a life where someone could be focused more or less entirely on what's going on with them in a given moment difficult to even imagine. I felt happy for Dan that that's his reality, and discovering that about him offered me a little insight into how other people's minds operate, a topic that would become fascinating to me over the coming months.

The next morning I was off again, out of Southampton and bounding towards the New Forest. I was a little fuzzy from the night before and decided that if I stood any chance of making it all the way around Britain I was probably going to have to ease up on the drinking and start getting all my kicks from nature. And what a place to start doing that . . .

The New Forest was established in the eleventh century by William the Conqueror as a place for him to hunt deer. Over the centuries, this 220-square-mile tract of forest, pasture and heathland has become home to thousands of species of plants, birds, reptiles and mammals, most notably the wild ponies, the New Forest groundskeepers, that roam freely and graze in the woodland and on the open heath. As I moseyed through I saw deer hurtling across stretches of trail ahead of me, then, along the north-eastern side of the forest, near Ashurst, the forest grows dense. Old and new trees fight for root space, thick canopies plunge the woodland into tracts of long and sinister shadows, clambering over uprooted trees and making the gnarled and twisted logs look like something out of a Tim Burton film. With the start of the South West Coast Path just a few days ahead of me, I knew it would be a long time until I was in woods like these again so I really made the most of it.

I followed the trail for ten miles towards a small village called Brockenhurst. Lots of the houses there have cattle grids at the end of their drives because the ponies like to saunter into town from the woods so they can buy fags. All right, they don't do that, but they do just wander into town whenever they feel like it, something that everyone who lives in that area seems pleasantly relaxed about.

At times I wished I had a bike – there are some great stretches of dirt track between Brockenhurst and New Milton that were a bit long and boring on foot – but still it was all very picturesque. I tried to remember some of the games Sam and I used to play in the woods when we were kids, how satisfying it was to cut down bracken and the excitement we felt when we found a *really* good stick. (You can't really describe a 'good stick'; it's more a feeling you get when you spot one, and when you pick it up you just know.)

I made relatively light work of the New Forest, covering the thirty or so miles between Southampton and Bournemouth in two days. It was easy to find nice spots to camp (although I'm pretty sure you're not supposed to, legally speaking) and there were plenty of creatures in the woods to keep me entertained as I passed through. I was getting more confident in my map-reading, and I was amazed at how far I was travelling by foot each day – it added up to almost a hundred miles by the time I'd reached the Dorset coast. Watching the landscape change mile by mile, step by step, in such detail, is a privilege, and one only really achievable when travelling on foot.

I'd soon be rejoining the coast. The sound of waves and the salty smell in the air had been distinctly lacking since my first day, when I walked to Worthing, and despite enjoying the downs, I realized deep down that I'd been missing the sea. Before going to Brighton to begin my journey, I hadn't been on the coast in a long time, and after a brief taste of it on that first day I was now craving it, which was just as well, as I'd soon be walking the South West Coast Path – a 630-mile national trail that would take me through the rugged coastlines of Dorset, South Devon, Cornwall, North Devon and Somerset. I saw it as a sort of challenge within a challenge, one that I had been looking forward to since I'd discovered the trail while plotting my journey.

After a damp, scrappy wade through the farmland and overgrown footpaths of the Avon Way I arrived on the shores of Bournemouth, ten days after leaving Brighton. Unlike the shingle beaches of my home from home, Bournemouth's is covered in fine, golden sand, so I indulged in a gentle barefoot potter along the strand.

Before setting off, I'd downloaded Couchsurfing, a social networking app that connects travellers looking for and those offering places to crash. I'd used it a few years previously while interrailing on my own around Europe and loved it; it was like having friends you never knew you had showing you around places you'd never been. I once couchsurfed with someone called Josefine in Malmö, Sweden, who, after a whistle-stop tour of the city's metal bars, took me to a Halloween party where a guy dressed as a post-crucified Jesus forcibly pierced my ear with a safety pin while I was going to the toilet. While having my flesh lanced by a punk dressed as Jesus wasn't exactly what I'd signed up for, I reasoned that if I was all right with walking blindly into a stranger's life, then I couldn't really get upset if anything weird happened while I was there. As convenient as finding a sofa to crash on can be, I was under no illusions that it can, on occasion, come with things I might not expect.

After finding some profiles in Bournemouth and Poole, I sent a few messages out into the Couchsurfing ether. It was the first time I'd used the app on home soil and, although an English stoner guy called Barney had put me up in Paris a few years previously, I was sceptical of how trusting and accommodating English people would be towards travellers in their own country. It was therefore little surprise that the

67

person who responded was someone called Oana, and her English had a non-English tint. She told me she lived in Poole and would be happy to put me up for the night. After stocking up on food supplies I took a slow walk along the seafront to her place and arrived there at around 6 p.m.

Oana was a Romanian travel blogger who, since Romania had entered the EU in 2007, had spent time in almost every country in Europe. She'd been living on the Dorset coast for two years after spending two years in Rome. She looked to me to be in her late twenties, which meant she'd been travelling for almost a third of her life, something that impressed me enormously and demonstrated that, like me, she was someone who valued new places and experiences. She suggested we take a walk down to the quay that overlooks Poole Harbour. The sun gradually fell towards the horizon and by the time we reached the quay the air was cool and the sky awash with oranges, reds and pinks. The silhouettes of fishing boats bobbing playfully around in the harbour made the reflected orange sunlight shimmer off the water like thousands of tiny flames. It was such a treat to get a feel for where I was, taking in my surroundings rather than just ploughing through.

I packed up and left early the next morning. After pointing out and impressively naming the small islands in the harbour the night before, Oana had pointed me in the direction of the Studland Peninsula, where the South West Coast Path begins. She told me I had to catch a toll ferry over to South Haven Point, and that the earliest one was at 7.10 a.m.

Walking towards Sandbanks to catch the ferry, I noticed that I felt a little sad to be leaving Poole. I think I'd probably got to know it slightly better than the other towns I'd stopped in, and something about being down on the quay at sunset, the smell of the water and the gentle clanging of masts in the wind had made me miss Maldon. I decided to message Mum to ask how she felt about coming out and joining me for a bit of the walk. She said she'd love to see some of the Cornish coast, and we agreed that we'd arrange her coming out when I got closer to Cornwall in a few weeks' time.

As the chains tightened and the ferry ground to a halt at South Haven Point, I took a moment to make sure we'd properly stopped. With a maximum speed of, I don't know, 1 mph?, the ferry is easily the least thrilling mode of transport I've ever used. Someone told me that it's Britain's most expensive mode of public transport in terms of the cost to distance travelled ratio, despite only being a quid. Once I alighted the ferry I began walking along the tarmac towards a curiously placed red telephone box some fifty yards ahead of me. It was an iconic red London one, not one of those Bob Hoskins 'Good to Talk' ones. I couldn't figure out why it was there, but I kind of liked that. It should have looked out of place, but it didn't, like a bow tie on a penguin.

My eyes wandered west and I clocked the beach. The Studland Peninsula is a really beautiful place. The sand's so bright and natural-looking and is dutifully watched over by a large band of dunes on its northern side. It's long and swings out like a scythe, and as the dunes peter out the land swells and you can just make out Dover's white-cliffed coastline.

The sand was irresistible, so I decided to walk the first mile of this monumental pathway barefoot. I took off my boots and fastened them to my pack using some bungee cords I'd liberated from the wheelhouse of Mum's boat. I thought about using my laces to secure them a little tighter but decided against it – the bungees looked sturdy enough.

As I got to my feet I felt a surge of energy. The warmth from the sun, the wind through my hair, that salty smell in the air, it all hit me at once, and as I began walking, the sand nestling between my toes, I entered a state of total natural euphoria. My body was in harmony with my surroundings and my mind was free of all worry. It was bliss.

I wandered along and, as I approached the end of the beach, maybe a mile or so from where it began, I noticed a small clearing in the bushes and the first of a set of steps which presumably led up to the cliffs, and headed towards them. The cliffs curved back in on themselves after about a hundred yards then disappeared around a corner. Maybe I could circle the base of the cliff and find a neighbouring beach – perhaps a secret beach that nobody had yet discovered. I checked my map and deciphered that this could well be the case – it's quite easy to see what you want to see on a map, even an Ordnance Survey one. I looked back towards the steps, scoffed, then pootled off towards the cliff base, blindly eager and convinced I'd made a truly brilliant decision.

The terrain underfoot turned to shingle almost immediately. It was jagged and quite painful to walk on, but instead of putting my boots back on I decided to wade through the water, which was only a little higher than ankle deep. The tide was coming in and a little further on I felt seaweed on my feet, and slippery stones, as the sand retreated further into the surf. The water now sat just above my knee. My initial excitable pace had slowed to a slightly self-conscious trudge, and as a wave approached and I got clumsily up on tiptoe to avoid the base of my pack getting wet I began to question my reasoning some fifteen minutes earlier, back at the steps.

I continued to wade, using my feet to scour the ground ahead of me as I could no longer see the bottom clearly through the water. After a few more steps I felt the wet hit my left bum cheek – the tide was coming in fast. With my hands stretched out in front of me, I turned towards the shore to see if there was still some shingle at the base of the cliff. Thankfully, there was, so I began wading towards the shore. The rocks got sharper beneath my feet the closer I got and by the time I made it to land I felt like I was walking on broken light bulbs. I hobbled towards a nearby rock, unclipped my pack and let it fall from my back on to the floor. I turned it over and, to my horror, saw that there was only one boot attached.

In a moment of hot, white panic, I felt around the pack, refusing to accept the obvious fact that one of them had slipped off while I was wading through the water. I spun around desperately to see where I'd walked from. The tide had risen even further, and pretty soon even the jagged floor beneath me would be completely submerged. I froze, my mouth open, staring blankly into nothing and holding my head between my hands like a vice, pushing tighter, as if squeezing it might force a solution into my frontal lobe. No such luck. On instinct, I waded unsteadily back into the sea, leaving my pack and single boot at the foot of the cliff, combing the water for my grey-and-black walking boot on a bed of grey-and-black rocks covered in almost black seaweed. It was hopeless. What I really needed was a pair of goggles. The second I thought this I dived under and began to swim as fast as I could back to the beach, acutely aware that the tide wasn't going to help me out in any way and that time was of the essence.

The water was so cold it took my breath away, but discomfort was way down my list of priorities. Back at the beach, I clambered out of the water with huge, sodden lunges. I honed in on a group of thirty-somethings who seemed pretty prepared for a day at the beach, thinking that somewhere in their hampers and day bags they might have what I needed.

I approached them, fully dressed, drenched and, I'm fairly certain, with a desperate look in my eyes.

'Guys, I'm sorry to interrupt but I'm in a real situation and I need a favour . . .' I gave them the shortest possible version of what had happened and ended up with: 'Does anyone have a pair of goggles I can borrow?'

'Yeah, man, I do,' said a tanned young man in sunglasses and red shorts. He reached into his bag, pulled them out and without hesitation, handed them to me.

I was so pathetically grateful. 'I'll bring them right back,' I promised, and marched back towards the sea, the lingering stare of the group hot on my back. I waded until my knees were submerged and dived in, staying underwater for a good seven or eight seconds, thinking it would be funny if the group thought I'd completely disappeared. I had to give them something.

While I was under I let go of all the stress of losing my boot for a moment. Swimming underwater is the only way I can really feel like I've entered another world, where everything is different, down to how my body moves. My mum decided she wanted to live on a boat because she has a deep need to live near water (or I guess on it in her case), and I think it's a need that we share. To me the sea is more than a healer, it's a life-giver, a physical presence full of power, mystery and life, and I'll be forever drawn to it.

After that moment came a feeling of crushing defeat. I'd lost my initial frustration and felt calmer, but that was annoying because my frustration had so far kept my motivation up. Now, I was slowly beginning to accept that my . . . *There it is!!* About twenty yards ahead of me, beneath the water, poking out from a rock, was my boot. I locked in on it and swam closer, a smile creeping on to my face as I realized that the ordeal was coming to an end; I'd be able to get back on track and enjoy the . . . Wait . . . Hang on . . . I grabbed the boot and stood up. I didn't even need to look at it. It wasn't my boot. It seemed some other dipshit had lost their boot in the exact same place as I had. I leaned back and, using all my weight, launched the dumb, rotting, honking, semi-lived-in crab's house as far away from me as I could.

'FUCKKK OFFFFF!!!!' I roared at it as it sailed through the air. It landed near the cliff base, some ten or so yards away. Even the plopping sound it made was irritating.

I stared out to sea for a few seconds then went back under the water. My watch told me I'd had the goggles for about forty minutes and I started to worry the bloke in the red shorts would think I'd made off with them, but I thought I'd keep trying a little bit longer before I had to admit defeat and return them.

I swam to the base of the cliffs where I'd left my rucksack. Nothing. I swam back towards the beach, staring at the sea-bed like an eagle hunting prey. Again, nothing. I swam out a little deeper, then headed back towards the cliffs once more. I'd had enough. I was tired, and I wasn't going to find it. I'd have to swim back to the beach to return the goggles any-way, I thought, so I might as well at least try and enjoy that. I sunk under the water and focused on doing the best breast-stroke I could, one where I could glide above the sand and the seaweed and the . . . *Oh my God, there it is!!!*

Nestled in the seaweed right ahead of me lay my trusty, dejected boot. No wonder I hadn't seen it before; it had sunk in so deep only the sole was visible. I couldn't believe it. I plucked it lovingly from its bed and hoisted myself out of the water. I held it up in front of me and my heart sank. It wasn't my boot. I'd rediscovered the one I'd found and thrown away earlier. I felt like crying. This time, I just let go of it and watched it sink down on to the seaweed, like Rose letting Jack go at the end of *Titanic*.

Traversing the jagged shingle in my bare feet to get my pack, I actually felt depressed. I picked up my pack and, as I did so, my other boot came free of the bungee cord and fell to the ground. I stared at it as I put my rucksack back on, then placed it on a nearby rock. When I returned the goggles, not many words were exchanged. There was no need. I'd come back empty-handed, still barefoot, looking sullen and dejected. To ask me how it went would have been as mean as laughing.

That night I slept on top of the cliffs right by Old Harry's Rocks, a really cool offshore chalk formation made up of three large precipices at Handfast Point on the Isle of Purbeck. It's probably the third most iconic feature of the Dorset coast, I'd say, after Lulworth Cove and Durdle Door and, feeling like I owed myself a little wonderment after my utter shambles of an afternoon, I decided to treat myself to a camp with a view. Before I went to sleep I used my map to locate the nearest place I could buy a pair of boots. I'd managed to walk up the many steps from the beach and on to the cliffs all right, but it hadn't taken long; I didn't want to walk miles with no boots. Thankfully, Swanage was only five or so miles along the coastal path.

'Five miles,' I thought to myself, and dived into my pack to check how many pairs of socks I had. Fours pairs of double-layered socks so eight pairs . . . kind of. I liberated two of the three plastic bags I'd packed for 'unforeseeable emergencies' and put them with my socks in a pile at the foot of the tent.

'That'll do, as long as it doesn't rain,' I reasoned, and lay down in my sleeping bag. It had been an exhausting day and I was asleep within minutes.

I woke in a daze. The wind had picked up at around eleven and kept me up for most of the night. The sound of the Flea being thrashed around was as loud and annoying as a trolley falling down a concrete fire escape. I made some mental notes:

Don't sleep on a clifftop again.
Buy earplugs.

I pulled the door aside, revealing thick grey clouds, long grass blowing maniacally in the wind and, of course, *rain*. I grabbed the pile of socks and bags I'd left for myself and one by one yanked them over my feet. Before the final sock, I popped the bags on. I stopped and stared at my feet for a moment.

I felt like such a knob. Here I was at the start of a 3,000-mile walk around the country, one that I was now thinking would probably take close to a year to complete, and within the first two weeks I'd lost my fucking boots.

My feet took an absolute pounding on the cliffs on the two-hour walk, and when I got into Swanage, at around 11 a.m., I was tired, wet and angry. I found Jurassic Outdoor, peered through the door and got the attention of the shop assistant by announcing, quite loudly: 'I'm gonna come in without shoes, OK? But I'm coming in specifically to *buy* shoes so whatever I buy I'll put them on, when I buy them.' The shop assistant stared back at me with the blankest expression I'd ever seen.

I clenched my jaw. 'I'm coming in,' I said, to nobody in particular. I squelched into the shop and made a beeline for the section that seemed to cater for the male walker. I picked up a boot I liked the look of and turned it over – a hundred and fifty quid. I placed it back on its little boot-sized plastic shelf gently, like it was a Fabergé egg or something, and carried on looking. I saw another pair that looked all right – sixty quid. That was better, and they would, after all, be with me on a walk all around Britain.

After an awkward minute or so where neither the shop assistant or I acknowledged that I was trying the boots on with visibly soaked socks, I bought them and left the shop. I checked into a hostel, another expense but a necessary one – to dry my socks, wash my clothes and take a hot shower. It had been a long twenty-four hours, and the most stressed I'd felt on the walk so far. It was important to me to feel like I'd put an end to the stress. I could start afresh the next day.

7

Over the following few days my new boots and I set about conquering the Jurassic coast. I didn't properly acknowledge it at the time, I don't think, but having the sea to my left every day meant I had constant access to something that not only relaxed me but allowed me to think clearly and even to ponder the future. Wallace J. Nichols, an American author and marine biologist, believes that humans have a 'blue mind' and that we achieve, as he puts it, 'a mildly meditative state characterized by calm, peacefulness, unity, and a sense of general happiness and satisfaction with life, when we're in or near water'. After the unprecedented stress of the whole lost-boot saga, it was probably fortunate that I'm as suscept-ible to the healing power of water as I am.

I continued west, following the wooden signposts that shepherd the coastal path. There's very little in the way of flat ground on the Jurassic Coast, which makes carrying your home and possessions around on your back like a snail an exhausting exercise at times. The route is a more or less con-stant stream of inclines and declines that follow one another successively like sound waves. The shifts in gradient made my thigh muscles burn deep and raw as I passed the various markers – Blackers Hole, Dancing Ledge, Seacombe Cliff – that cling to Dorset's blustery coast. It was hard work, but the good kind – the kind you know is making you stronger and getting you somewhere.

As I reached St Aldhelm's Head I checked my map: the upcoming section of coast was labelled: 'DANGER AREA'.

This, my friend Phil had explained to me during our pre-walk map-reading lesson, generally means that a particular section of land or space is being used by the MOD for manoeuvres, and if this is signalled by a red flag, then there's absolutely no way of getting through it. I decided that rather than follow the coastal path as far as I could before changing course I would head inland early via a narrow side path, through the village of Kingston and towards the ruins of Corfe Castle, which, along with the New Forest, was the second lasting emblem of William the Conqueror I'd come across that fortnight.

Britain's great for castle-spotting. Although most of them are now ruins, they still loom proudly along our shores, especially in the north-east, on the Northumberland coast. Throughout my walk I developed a real affinity for them, and any site of historical significance, for that matter. They offer a glimpse into a time and a way of life that's almost impossible to imagine, yet the natural surroundings would have been more or less the same then as they are today.

It was getting late and the clouds that had been sitting so harmlessly overhead for the best part of the afternoon were beginning to darken, and the time had come to think about where I could set up camp for the night.

Wild camping can be tricky in England as most of the countryside is privately owned by farmers, the National Trust or families descended from aristocracy. Even if you turn up late, leave early and leave your plot exactly how you found it, there's always a chance you'll (quite rightly) have to contend with an exasperated landowner demanding to know what 'the hell you think you're doing' on their land, and factoring in that my thus far dependable National Trust coast path was being used for target practice that evening, I was left trawling field after field, hedgerow after hedgerow, hoping to come across a secluded spot where I wouldn't get hassled. After an hour or so I was forced to widen the search beyond the landmass itself and began to include people in my hunt. This was how I ended up meeting and spending the night with Robbie.

I bumped into Robbie on a quiet B-road two or so miles west of Corfe Castle. He was a rustic local in his mid- to late-fifties, a slender man with shaggy dark hair and rosy time-worn skin. His thick wax coat and savagely overworked wellington boots sandwiched a beaten-up pair of cream cords. He was, by all visible accounts, a true countryman and, apart from a pair of dotty old dears I'd got chatting to near the castle, he was also the only human I'd managed to meet head-on in about twenty minutes. With time getting on, my scope to seek help from a local was becoming limited.

'Hi, mate,' I said, approaching him.

'Oh, hello,' he replied. His eyes were grey and kind and his tone was neighbourly. I could tell immediately he was a good guy.

'I'm just looking for a place to camp – I can't pitch anywhere on the coast path because of the –'

'Yes, they're firing off rounds out there tonight, I believe.'

'Yes, exactly. I've been searching, but it looks like everywhere round here's private land. I don't suppose you know anywhere near here, do you? Or someone who wouldn't mind me using their field for the night?'

Too obvious?

'How far are you heading?'

'Well, I walked here from Brighton,' I said. 'I'm doing the whole trail round to Minehead.'

At this point I was only telling people that I was walking the South West Coastal Path, rather than all around Britain. Considering the inordinate mileage I still had ahead of me, it just seemed more believable, and still seemed pretty impressive.

'Wow,' said the man. 'That's pretty impressive . . . Well, like you said, there isn't much by way of decent camping spots round here, but you're very welcome to pitch up in my garden if you like. I only live about ten minutes away.'

My initial gratitude and relief quickly turned into a buzz, like I'd just been invited to an impromptu party in the woods. I leaned in to shake the man's hand.

'I'm Jake, by the way.'

'Robbie,' said Robbie. He extended a hand and his eyes danced as he looked at me. Good vibes turned great; I knew Robbie was going to become my friend.

Robbie was only the second stranger to invite me into their home and, much like the Browns, who had asked me to dinner a week or so previously, Robbie appeared to relish the chance to host a drifter. His house was a beautiful old grey stone cottage that sat quietly at the edge of the woods, complete with cabinets full of interesting trinkets and worn, crooked rooms bedecked with lived-in furniture. Over the course of the evening he put together a homey spread of food, ran me a bath and dutifully kept my glass topped up while we took it in turns to introduce each other to the music we liked. It really was a sterling hosting effort from Robbie.

It takes a certain type of person to go to that much effort to accommodate an outsider – a lot of trust and benevolence, obviously, but an above-averagely inquiring mind too, I think. In much the same way that hitchhikers are most likely to be picked up by people who are like them – usually other hitchhikers – I was beginning to notice subtle similarities between the people who invited me into their homes: threads of openness, intrigue and trust that bound them together, regardless of age, nationality or gender. At the end of the evening Robbie upgraded his offer of a pitch for the Flea in his garden and offered me the spare room.

The following morning, over a few rounds of bacon and eggs and lashings of hot tea, Robbie and I shared a few frivolities, and then I was gone. I remember thinking how strange it was that I'd likely never see him again, maybe never even speak to him again. That's not necessarily what I wanted; it just felt like that's how it would be with anyone I met in this new, transient life. There was something both sad and unfettering about it, a sense of 'That was brilliant, and now it's time to move on.' Usually when I establish a proper connection with somebody I really don't want to let it go. Those connections, like the one I had with Robbie, are rare, and my natural instinct has always been to try and hang on to people I connect with on that sort of level. The fact that I found it easy to leave Robbie's without feeling like I was abandoning something special had to be down to my current life being so different, everything now so temporary. I wasn't quite aware of it then, but even feelings and emotions that I'd normally dwell on were passing quickly, and as I set off that morning my focus switched straight back to the road ahead of me, to the mystery and uncertainty of what lay ahead.

I headed west along the ridge overlooking Church Knowle for maybe an hour before I was forced to change course. It ran right into the MOD's 'DANGER AREA', and the quickest way around it I could see on the map was via a trail called the Hardy Way. As I already had my phone out, I took the opportunity to see if the trail had a story. I discovered that it's fairly new, created in the 1990s by a walking enthusiast called Margaret Marande, who devised a long-distance footpath that links some of the locations described in the novels and poems of Thomas Hardy, of whom she was clearly quite the fan. I remember wishing that I'd thought to look into the origins of some of the trails I'd be walking on in advance, and maybe brought a book by Hardy to read as I walked the pathway dedicated to him. That said, I also had to remind myself that, as enjoyable as this walk was becoming, I had to remain focused on why I was doing it.

The Hardy Way is marked by distinctive green discs nailed to wooden posts, which led me as far north as the village of Stoborough. From there I continued west, along the top of the DANGER AREA, until I reached a point where I could head south, back towards the coast. After a few more hours I reached Lulworth Cove. I gazed in awe from the water's edge; sheets of grass on the surrounding hills pour over the tops of the white chalk cliffs and encircle the water like green lava, with a gap in the limestone at the mouth of the cove that acts as a doorway to the sea beyond. It's as tranquil and majestic a place as you're likely to encounter on England's south coast. Just a few hundred yards along from Lulworth Cove is Durdle Door, an iconic limestone arch that gazes boldly over the beach. I had a hazy childhood memory of being there before, me and my brother throwing stones into the sea, barely aware of the stunning scenery that surrounded us.

My walk to and past these landmarks signified my return to the South West Coast Path and, as a treat for getting back on track, I lumbered down the crooked steps to Durdle Door beach, shed my pack and everything but my shorts and dived into the sea. The water wasn't too cold, and after I'd sub-merged myself entirely I swam out as far as I could under water, not surfacing until I needed air. Soaking up the sun all day and cooling off my skin and aching muscles in the water felt so leisurely, like being on holiday. I was feeling fit and strong and in a really good place mentally, not worrying about how long I'd be walking, distance or time, or question-ing my decision to live in this way for the however many months that lay ahead. For once, I was just in the moment, enjoying the feeling of being. That night I camped on a hill near Osmington and had the best night of tent sleep I'd had so far.

Despite losing my boots, being hung-over a bit too often and getting lost occasionally, my first two weeks on the road felt like they'd been successful. I'd found my stride – but the best thing was that I felt happy. There was still a lot of excite-ment about it all – this new lifestyle, discovering different places and the satisfaction of looking at the map every day to see how far I'd walked. In the most positive sense, it didn't feel like me who was out there; it felt more like I was watch-ing someone else, someone living the perfect life. I felt like as long as I kept just plodding along, enjoying feeling fit and healthy, leaving myself open-minded enough to fall into unpredictable situations, I was going to be happy – a feeling that not so long ago I was convinced I'd never experience again.

I was also building up a decent-looking tan, which made me realize that it had been a long while since I'd felt remotely happy with my appearance. When I was living in east Lon-don I felt repulsed whenever I caught my reflection; I was pale, puffed up and had huge heavy bags under my eyes all the time. Not hating how I looked was definitely a sign that things had got better. But most of all I loved the feeling of being outside all the time. I loved waking up and realizing I was just in some field somewhere; I loved unzipping my tent door and listening to the birds; I loved how walking through leaves released their aroma; I loved always catching the first star in the sky at night; I loved how, no matter how many miles I walked and how tired I got, I never regretted doing it. Those 120 miles from Brighton to Durdle Door had given me a lot more than just a wholesome distraction from depression; they had made me feel grateful and happy to be alive. The days were getting warmer, and there was no need to rush anything.

The only thing that did concern me, on occasion, was the thought of getting injured. Over the following days I stuck vigilantly to the coastal path and discovered that walking across cliff tops all day is tough. As each day went on, the hills would feel more and more challenging, which was fine if there was just the one steep gradient per day, but the Jurassic Coast is a more or less constant stream of ups and downs, and it wasn't long before my legs were feeling the pinch. Most nights I found myself waking up with a general dull ache and had to improvise some stretches for my thighs and calves in my sleeping bag before I could go back to sleep.

I kept thinking that if the challenge got derailed because I picked up an injury that could have been avoided, I'd have no one to blame but myself, and I couldn't bear the thought of the people back home laying on the sympathy – 'Chin up, son, I couldn't have done much better' – so I began stretching every morning and, after reading about how swimming in cold water can aid recovery, I took a swim in the sea most evenings.

As the days went on and the path continued to ascend and descend on the clifftops, I noticed I was feeling physically stronger. My legs had become hardened and muscular, my back, too, and it wasn't long before I'd puffed and sweated the entire forty-mile stretch of coast between West Lulworth and Lyme Regis. I was about to hit Devon, the fifth county I'd be walking through, after East and West Sussex (definitely two counties), Hampshire and Dorset. I'd been walking for not quite a month, and as the white cliffs turned a dusty red it was the first time I actually considered the passing of time – and it became clear that I was going to be walking for longer than my originally planned seven months. But I felt so detached from a life where time had any impact that it was difficult to imagine ever wishing hours and weeks away, giving myself deadlines and time frames and pretending that any of it mattered.

I traversed the Devon coastline with the sea to my left until I reached Branscombe. It seemed like I hadn't seen a cloud in weeks and, although I felt good in myself, the heat was beginning to get to me. In most other scenarios I'd have called it 'perfect Calippo weather', but walking in it for miles under the weight of a twenty-kilo rucksack was often uncomfortable. I'd been dotting inland once a day to charge my phone and fill up my water bottles but, despite drinking upwards of six litres of water a day, there wasn't a lot of pee-ing going on, a sure sign that my body was using up every drop to help cool me down. I had to be careful with my skin, too, being extra vigilant with the factor 30 and making sure I wore a cap to shield my face.

The evenings were balmy and still enough for me to camp right on the beach, where the sound of waves sent me off into uninterrupted eight-hour slumbers. I woke early every morning, refreshed and motivated to take on the barrage of steep ascents that I sensed would keep coming as I approached Cornwall, and set off on what ended up being interminable days of ups, downs, craggy pathways and swollen knees. The red cliffs of Devon seemed even longer, steeper and more numerous than their white Dorset counterparts and, with the sun beating down relentlessly, there were times I genuinely thought I might pass out.

I made a decision to break away from the coastal path for a spell, partly to get some shade, but also just to change my route up. (I tend to get incredibly bored of anything repetitive after a while.) I'd met an American girl called Stacey just outside Torquay who had taken two months off work to fly to England and, as she put it, 'just start walking'. I suggested we head inland for a day or two so she could get a feel for an English town that wasn't all about buckets and spades and 99s.

Stacey, seemingly quite chuffed to have some company, was happy to go with it, so we ducked inland and made our way west to Totnes, a small town in South Devon that claims, rather outrageously, to be twinned with Narnia. After three or four hours we found ourselves passing through a track lined with people with dreadlocks living in vans – it seemed we were close. Apparently recognizing our collective need for one, Stacey suggested we find a proper campsite in town where we could shower and treat ourselves to fully functioning toilets – a suggestion I'd come to hugely appreciate over the following days.

The day before, worried I might be in danger of dehydrating, I'd filled my water bottles from a stream, taking what felt like my first opportunity to act like a true outdoorsman. However, without water-purifying tablets or any real knowledge of how to identify safe natural drinking water, I had rolled the dice on whether my Bear Grylls moment would simply quench my thirst or end up giving me the shits. After arriving in Totnes and finding a campsite I noticed I felt poorly, and not just normal poorly, really poorly – far from the comfort of a house, bed and bathroom poorly. Diarrhoea, we can probably all agree, is an unpleasant experience in most settings, but having diarrhoea when you're living in a tent is about as miserable as it gets. I spent that night waking up every hour and a half in a hot, sweaty panic and hurriedly clenching my way over to the campsite toilets. My plight continued way into the morning, until about nine o'clock, when Stacey came knocking. 'I don't feel very well,' I whimpered through the mesh, before giving her a brief sum-up of my bowel movements.

Stacey insisted on going into town to pick up some food for me. While she was gone I remembered that my friend Matt from back home had offered to pay for some accommodation if I ever needed it, and after a chat on the phone (he found my situation greatly amusing) he booked me into a local bed and breakfast. What a hero.

When Stacey returned I thanked her for coming back but insisted that she keep moving; I couldn't stand up straight, let alone walk, and she only had a few more weeks before she had to fly home. Plus, the thought of unzipping my tent fully and releasing the smell of a night's worth of risky farting would almost certainly break our, thus far, very relaxed rapport. We exchanged numbers, and cash for the snacks, then she left. We stayed in touch by text for a week or so afterwards, with the obligatory 'we must hook up again before you fly back' pleasantries, but that morning would be the last time I saw her.

I stayed in the B&B that Matt hooked me up with for two nights. The whole ordeal had set me back and made me feel weak, so it was with a heavy heart and a sore arse that I decided that the right move was not to go back on to the cliffs, but to travel the twenty-four miles I would have walked to Plymouth, had I been in a fit state, by train. From there I'd walk to Devil's Point and take the ferry across the River Tamar, to Cremyll, as planned, and continue walking the coastal path into Cornwall from there. I was kicking myself for hopping on a train because, even though I was ill, I couldn't help but feel like I'd cheated. For the first time since the walk began, the wheels were beginning to feel a little loose.

Arriving in Cornwall, however, gave me a lift. It's a section of Britain I'd always wanted to explore fully and now, finally, here I was, with a tent and a sleeping bag on my back and nothing but hundreds of miles of coastline ahead of me. Cornwall is so different to anywhere else in Britain that it's still considered by some (mostly Cornish people) to be the fifth country in the United Kingdom. It does kind of have its own feel, its own way of life, and I was looking forward to experiencing Cornish hospitality first hand.

I stuck religiously to the South West Coast Path, camping at Rame Head, where I was woken up by wild ponies first thing in the morning, then past Penlee Point, through the villages of Seaton and Polperro.

Polperro was stunning – a charming little fishing village, and one of the few places I earmarked as a possible place to live once the walk was over. I hadn't thought much about what I was going to do afterwards, at least not in any more detail than 'I can see me living here, drinking in that nice little boozer.' Thinking about my future felt almost reductive, like it pulled focus away from how much I was enjoying the present. I felt happier than ever while I was walking that section of the Cornish coast, so happy that my energy felt boundless.

Three days later, I'd walked a further fifty miles of coastline, and was about to enter Coverack, a village ten or so miles north of the Lizard Peninsula.

I located a pub, went in and bought a lime and soda then parked myself next to the only socket I could find so that I could charge my phone. In a corner of the room there was a pool table, where a couple of young lads were playing. One of them had what I considered to be a fairly classic Cornwall look – shaggy, salty hair, an incredible tan, denim shorts and an oversized flannel shirt, the kind of nineties grunge look I liked. The other was paler and scraggier. He wore a black cap, a black T-shirt and black jeans. He was clearly hammered, much to the amusement of his sun-bleached friend. I had a feeling they'd start talking to me the second I sat down.

Up close, I could see they were probably in their early twenties – surfers, hitchhikers, the type of people I'd been hoping to hang out with in Cornwall. And thankfully, if you're walking around Britain and folks notice the enormous pack on your back, you can very easily get into a conversation with whoever you like. I used to love watching people's reactions when I told them I'd walked to wherever we were from Brighton – eyes widen, mouths open, bodies lean in; I guess everyone's interested to get to know someone who's doing something with their life that goes a little against the grain.

They introduced themselves as Tom (surfer) and Dave (pissed).

'What's with the rucksack?' asked Dave, slurring a bit.

Tom laughed quietly and wiped beer off his chin. 'Where are you trying to get to?' he said.

'The Lizard Peninsula,' I said. 'I figured it'd look great at sunset.'

'You'll never make it there in time for sunset today,' Dave interjected.

'Yeah, you should stay with us tonight then go in the morning. It'll be dark by the time you get there if you carry on today,' Tom said.

It was easily the quickest leap from 'hello' to 'you can stay with me' I'd encountered so far, but I had a good feeling about these two and decided then and there that if anyone ever offered me a place to crash for a night while I was on this journey, I just had to accept.

The two downed what was left of their beers and stood up, and the three of us left the pub and began walking back into Coverack, stopping off at the local chippie to grab some food en route. Coverack's an attractive place, in the way almost all seaside towns are. All the action is on the seafront, where small cafés and eateries sit neatly in a row, facing out towards the water. It was about 4 p.m. and the sun was still high in the sky. It seemed like it would be a really nice place to live.

'How far's the house?' I asked after a couple of minutes. Knowing that the day's walking was coming to an end had made my legs feel tired.

'It's not a house, it's a caravan,' Tom said. 'Just up here.'

'Ah, OK,' I said, pretending not to be at all phased that these guys were in fact travellers.

My lifetime lack of contact with travellers made my brain automatically latch on to everything negative I'd ever heard about them – untrustworthy, unpredictable, violent, etc. My gut, however, was telling me that these guys were all right and that their offer to put me up came from a place of kindness and respect, so as we turned off the main road and headed towards a car park where three or four caravans were, quite clearly, illegally stationed, my brain and my gut were locked in an argument about whether this was a good idea or a terrible one.

'The council have been trying to move us on for about four years. Never happens, so we just stay here.'

I liked his attitude.

As we entered the one caravan that had its door open I heard the voices of two other people coming from inside. I lumbered up the step and in through the door and found a couple more scraggly Cornwall types sitting on the sofa smoking a joint.

'Who's this?' one of them asked.

'This is Jake. He walked here from Brighton, he's gonna crash with us tonight,' Tom replied.

'Cool,' the other guy mumbled, not needing any more information than that, apparently.

In that second I felt he thought I was one of them, a traveller without conventional roots. That, or he was too high to bother following up on his original question. Either way, I felt strangely welcome.

The inside of the caravan smelt like fag ash and dog hair. The floor and all the surfaces were littered with clothes, beer cans and empty wine bottles and a veil of dust hung weightlessly in the air, made all the more visible by the solid stream of light that beamed through the front door as the sun began to set. I liked these guys but, honestly, I wasn't exactly stoked to be crashing on the floor or wherever it was they were planning on stuffing me for the night. One or two more people showed up as twilight set in, each bursting in with higher volume than the last.

My phone had died, it was beginning to get dark and for some reason nobody had thought to turn a light on. As the minutes went by and the caravan was plunged into darkness, being too polite to ask why nobody was turning on a light, I went straight into worst-case-scenario thinking. *Why don't they want people to see us? Why did that guy who turned up last not introduce himself and then look at me weird? Why is everyone OK with not being able to see what's going on in here?*

Eventually, I had to ask. 'Sorry, mate, I don't suppose I could chuck a light on, could I?'

'The genny's out of diesel. Dave's mum went out to get some hours ago but she's not back yet.'

Dave's *mum*?!

I'd been so convinced that this lot lived here on their own the thought of there being a responsible adult on the scene came as a bit of a shock. I immediately felt sorry for Dave's mum. Clearly, this rabble of twenty-somethings had at one point overpowered her and taken control: if they wanted people round, they'd have people round; and if it's a mess, it's a mess; and if the generator runs out of diesel, it's all good because Mum can always nip out and buy some more. I instinctively started feeling around for empty beer cans and pushing them into a pile, trying not to make it too obvious I was having a bit of a tidy.

A few minutes later a car pulled up and the caravan was briefly lit up by the orange glow of dipped headlights.

'Dave, your mum's here,' someone said.

Dave got up and went to the door. I thought for a second that, with his mum being back and there being a bit of light from her headlights while she refilled the generator, they might have sprung into action and done something about the detritus, but no. I sat up and got myself ready to introduce myself to Dave's poor, downtrodden mum, maybe help her with the shopping, if she had any. The door burst open.

'Thisssfucjkingcuntjiussmuggedmeofffupbythefckkinn!'
Jesus.

'All right, Nancy!' The group seemed genuinely excited that she was home, and to hear what she was swearing so outrageously about.

'Who's this?' Nancy said, looking at me with a glassy, drunken stare.

'Sorry, I'm Jake. Sorry.'

'He's doing a big walk for mental health, Mum. He's staying here tonight,' said Dave.

'Mental health? I've got mental health,' said Nancy.

'Oh?' I said.

I often hear people say things like 'I suffer from mental health' or 'I've got mental health'; it's like the terminology isn't clear enough, so some people assume that mental health and mental illness are the same thing, which they aren't. While not everyone will at some point suffer from a mental illness – essentially a condition of the mind that requires treatment – everybody has mental *health*. If you have ever been happy, sad, excited, terrified, pissed off, etc., you have mental health, in the same way that if you have a heart, a brain, lungs, kidneys, legs, you have physical health.

I was too tired and a little overwhelmed by it all to remember afterwards what Nancy told me about herself that night, but I left the following morning with a feeling that it didn't matter. What our chat told me was that my life was so vastly different to hers, yet in the misery that life sometimes creates for us we found common ground. It's the feeling itself that people can relate to, so articulating depression in terms of the pain can sometimes help create the connection people need when nobody else is able to relate to the circumstances that led to it. I left Coverack with a renewed opinion about travellers. Obviously, this one experience with a few individuals doesn't sum an entire community up, but Tom, Dave and the rest of the gang did something for me that 99 per cent of people would never do – put up a total stranger for the sake of it, just to be decent. That, to me, says everything I need to know about a person.

I arrived at the Lizard Peninsula later that day and, just as Tom and Dave had promised, it was far more impressive than it would have been if I'd arrived after dark. That said, it was a bit of a tourist trap, which, as snobby as it sounds, put me off sticking around too long. That was OK, though. I wanted to push on because my friend Casey had been in touch to say he was visiting his parents, fifteen miles away in Helston, the following day. I hadn't spent any time with an actual friend since staying at Dan's in Southampton; for my own sanity, I had to make the effort to see my mates whenever I had a chance.

I haven't really ever been part of one specific really tight-knit group of friends, I've always floated around a few different groups, preferring, I suppose, to focus on one-on-one friendships. I often go long periods of time without really chatting to people I'd consider to be my best and oldest friends – I suppose I prefer low-maintenance friendships, keeping expectations nice and manageable. Sometimes, seeing friends I haven't seen in a while can make me anxious. I hate that, and at the time it kind of feels like I'm sabotaging my own opportunity to have a good time. But I know there's no controlling my social anxiety, and it helps to remind myself of that when I feel I'm a bit off – not that that ever seems to matter to my friends. At the end of the day, there's being anxious, which I can't control, and there's beating myself up for not being on top form, which I can. It's easier to get over being a bit quiet or less comfortable than usual if I treat myself with the same logic and understanding as my friends do. On this occasion, though, there was none of that. I felt relaxed, good in myself and excited to see Casey.

Casey and I met through playing music. We were introduced when a mutual friend of ours was recruiting for his band, a Brighton-based post-hardcore outfit called This City that was signed to the punk label Epitaph, back in 2008. Casey was being sized up to be the band's new drummer and, while my main instrument is guitar, This City were looking for a replacement bass player. After a few practice sessions Casey and I were recruited ahead of a three-week UK tour supporting new-rave outfit Hadouken! The band didn't know it at the time, but it would be my first live performance with a band since my excruciating debut at my Year 6 leaving assembly. My first-ever fully amplified gig was a pre-tour warm-up at The Garage in north London, where we were on a bill with two bands that were on the verge of hitting it big, Young Guns and You Me At Six. I posed awkwardly with a bass guitar I had to borrow off a mate the day before the show, but some of the bands that have performed on that stage could be considered some of the all-time giants of rock – Oasis, Red Hot Chili Peppers, Muse, Arctic Monkeys and Green Day. Thankfully, I did all right, and after three weeks of equally packed shows around the UK with Hadouken! I'd found my stage confidence and, through the excitement of feeling like we'd 'made it', Casey and I became close friends.

While being in a band is a lifestyle I've since moved away from, it's one where Casey has continued to thrive. He was playing drums for veteran emo outfit Funeral for a Friend at the time I was due to stay with him, and I considered it pretty lucky to catch him away from his relentless touring schedule. I spent a couple of days with him, and he seemed excited to host me in his home town. We spent most of our time in his local, drinking local beer, talking to the locals. It was all very . . . local. For all the catching up we did, my reasons for doing the walk never really came up. It seemed Casey and I were both doing well mentally at the time, so the need to 'get deep' never presented itself. When a friend knows you well, and knows that you sometimes get low but doesn't ask you how you are, it can be a good thing. Sometimes I'm not too sure how I am, and silent confirmation from a mate can help me see things for how they really are.

I'd had to come slightly inland to get to Helston, so once I'd said goodbye to Casey it was a quick couple of miles back to the fishing town of Porthleven so I could rejoin the coastal path. Mum had been in touch a week or so before I got to Cornwall. She'd been checking in on me fairly regularly, asking me to send her pictures of where I was and asking if I'd met any 'nice animals' – her little way of seeing if I'm all right. If I respond playfully with something like 'I've got three spiders living in my tent and they're all called Graham,' she knows I'm all right; if I don't respond at all, she knows something's up and usually follows up with a phone call. It was a good system and, mercifully, there hadn't been much need for those phone calls so far. She was keen to come out and join me for a section of my walk, as was my brother, Sam, for a second time. I noticed that my challenge was beginning to involve some deftness in time management and, in making plans to see people, organizing my time had, on occasion, got a little complicated. I was on top of it, though, kind of, and I suggested that Mum and Sam meet me at a point of some significance. I was about to change trajectory after walking west for the past month and a half, so Land's End felt like a fitting place to have some of my family with me.

I suggested meeting in Penzance, a day's walk from Helston, finding a campsite close to the coast and spending two days on the coastal path, bussing it back to the campsite at the halfway point. Mum liked the idea – she loves a good, solid plan – and when I arrived in Penzance two days after leaving Coverack there she was, all ready to go. Although I was doing OK with making and sticking to plans, it has to be said that Mum and my sister, Frank, are the organized people in my family. In comparison, Sam, my dad and I are, historically, pretty useless. So while Mum turned up on time, raring to go, sporting a recently purchased pair of walking boots and clutching a second-hand tent she'd bought on eBay the previous week, we had to sit and wait on Sam for four hours in some rotten old pub in Penzance town centre while he hitchhiked from Peckham clutching a tote bag.

We found a small campsite on the outskirts of Penzance, near Madron. We camped in a triangle and Mum and Sam laughed at how bad the Flea smelt. The following morning we got back on the coastal path, passing through Paul and Mousehole before the path led us back on top of the huge, prehistoric precipices that guard the land, cloaked with bright green grass and purple heather. It looked so perfect, and the sea looked colossal, like it could drown a planet. Now, I was no longer looking at the Channel between England and France, I was looking *out* out, into the Celtic Sea and, beyond that, the ocean. I thought about the hordes of people I'd seen swarming the Lizard Peninsula the week before and how much more beautiful the empty sections of coast Mum, Sam and I were passing through looked in comparison. The three of us walked fifteen miles from Penzance over two days, powering through the numerous inclines, declines, coves and clifftops, until around four in the afternoon on the second day, when we spied Land's End in the distance. I felt a rush, like the feeling you get when you see a friend you haven't seen in a long time, and as we got closer the magnitude of what was happening began to sink in. It had been forty-nine days since I'd left Brighton, and reaching Britain's most south-westerly point marked a huge milestone in my challenge: after over six weeks walking west through five counties and across hundreds of miles of exquisite English coastline, I had officially run out of land, and it would soon be time to start heading north.

I've never really had that gushing sense of victory that I notice some people have, the instinct to celebrate after achieving a 'goal'; so, in all honesty, reaching Britain's most southerly tip wasn't a punch-the-air moment. There were a few seconds, though, maybe a mile from Land's End, where what I was doing and how far I'd come really came into focus and I felt proud. The stretch of coast between Porthcurno and Land's End had been exquisite, and sharing it with Mum and Sam is something I'll remember forever.

After our time together, Mum wrote a blog and posted it online.

The two days I spent walking with Jake opened my eyes to the physical and mental endurance test he was undertaking as an antidote to the years of mismanaged stress which led to his depression. The term 'burn-out' was the best term to use to describe the symptoms my oldest son was experiencing when he called me one morning in March 2016, in tears, telling me how bad things were for him and how scared he felt for his own safety. His thoughts about everything were negative and bleak, his self-esteem and confidence had taken a huge hit and he was completely overwhelmed. *The only solution he could see to this was to work harder and longer to try to get on top of a situation he had already lost control of. When others, including his bosses, suggested that he took his foot off the gas and worked fewer hours, he dismissed this as impossible, fearful that things would run further and further from his grasp. Jake had given up all of the things that kept him happy and well in his quest to prove his worth: playing music, seeing friends, following football, eating good food, being outside (he didn't look like he had seen the sun for months) and his mood had spiralled downwards as a result.*

The man that came home after resigning from his job was withdrawn and lost. He spent the first couple of weeks licking his wounds and living very gently – not going out much, not drinking, sleeping a lot, occasionally cooking for us, and starting to exercise again as he slowly started to regain interest in such things. One day I came home from work and found him immersed in a map of the UK and he told me he'd had an idea that he was going to start walking. I didn't take it too seriously, but I was glad to see some of the lost enthusiasm and spark returning to him. Over the next four weeks, as the crowdfunding donations came pouring in, along with the hundreds of messages of kindness, identification, support and encouragement, things really started to change. Jake had rediscovered a purpose.

The Jake who was waiting for me at Penzance station, seven weeks and 350 miles into his mammoth 3,000-mile walk, looked like a strapping Danish backpacker; sun-bleached blond hair, tanned skin and a strong, muscular body (albeit there being 10 kg less of him since I last saw him). I hardly recognized him. He told me he loved his life now and appreciated so many things that he didn't have any time for before. He was learning to take setbacks in his stride and not allowing negative thoughts to take over when things go wrong. He was beginning to accept the fact that things wouldn't always go his way and that he wouldn't always like the way things are, but that nothing ever stays the same for long. He had lost his initial suspicion of strangers who show unexpected kindness (taking him to their homes to feed and water him and even provide a soft bed for the night) and as a result was no longer missing the good in people, which was not easy for him to see before. He had learned that setting small, achievable goals every day gave him a consistent sense of achievement and satisfaction which was rebuilding his self-confidence and sense of self-mastery. He knew that when he had pushed himself too far and imposed needless pressure on himself he needed to take a pause and think what is necessary to restore himself to balance.

Don't get me wrong – essentially, Jake is still the same person, with all the qualities and flaws that make him who he is. Seven weeks in a tent hadn't converted him into an expert, well-organized, outdoor type – he was still rolling his tent up wet, had lost a number of essential pieces of equipment, occasionally got lost and had maintained a significant Doritos habit.

Jake has never been the sort of person who wants to be told the best way to do things by those that think they know. Instead he learns by his own experience and then tries to work out what it is he has discovered. When you look at all the elements of this momentous walk – the exercise, the openness to others, a new appreciation of the small, simple things, the sense of achievement and purpose, the fresh air, the deep restorative sleep that comes with all of this – it's a manual to mental health that has been written about and endorsed by mental health professionals for years. In mental health jargon, it's an eclectic approach which includes Behavioural Activation, Mindfulness, CBT and Solution Focused Therapy. It doesn't matter to Jake what it's called. He found his own way and has continued leading by example – by inspiring young people who aren't interested in labels and theories but who just want to know how to feel better on those days when they don't want to get out of bed.

Needless to say, I am hugely proud of Jake, and also now impressed with the reality of what he is doing. Two days walking the South West Coastal Path was challenging, painful at times, breathtaking and *satisfying, but doing that day after day for months takes something that I don't think I've got. Something I certainly haven't taught Jake, but something that I am in awe of.*

She's very wise, my ma . . .
But I do *not* have a Doritos habit.

8

Back on my own again, I made relatively light work of the Cornish section of the South West Coast Path. The awesome cliffs and fields that sit atop kept me away from civilization for days, so when I passed through St Ives I once again found myself feeling slightly disappointed to be barging through swathes of sunburnt holiday-makers. That said, I still had to charge my phone and fill my water bottle up every day, and in every pub I went in to do this I was greeted with a curiosity and a warmth that felt distinctly Cornish. It wasn't uncommon for people to buy me a beer, sometimes even lunch. Cornwall appeared to have this amazing open-door policy; people simply couldn't do enough for me, especially when they found out why I was doing the walk. Depression had long convinced me that I wasn't worthy of genuine friendships, that I didn't deserve to experience genuine moments with people, but although I was on my own most of the time, flying solo along the Cornish coast is when I began to feel more sociable, more willing to be myself and to connect.

I pushed on, past the chapel ruins near Wheal Coates and across a deserted Poly Joke beach. The weather was turning and, having spent the last month in the sun, I became aware I had almost run out of summer and had only covered around four hundred miles of southern England. But time was only an issue if I allowed it to be. Since losing my boot and having to fork out for a new pair in Swanage, I'd been keeping to a revised budget of £15 a day and I felt like I had enough money and the right equipment to see me through the autumn and winter months. I also had purpose and patience, which an old, wiry gentleman who stopped me one day confirmed by referring to me as a 'King Arthur'. The man claimed to have discovered Excalibur underneath his kitchen floor thirty years ago and was now on a quest to locate the remaining 52,000 'King Arthurs' that are alive today. In his terms, a 'King Arthur' is a person on a quest that takes a lifetime to complete. Only they have the patience to achieve their ultimate goal in life, and I guess after I'd given him a run-down of what I was doing with my time, I fitted the brief. I was beginning to run into some very interesting characters on the Cornish coast.

The following evening, after a tiring fifteen miles, I stopped to take a look at my map. A man, probably in his sixties, was sat on a bench some twenty yards from me. He was tall and broad, with a face like a weathered rock. He was smoking a – frankly – enormous spliff and clutching a can of Tribute, the local tipple. He noticed me looking and muttered something under his breath. Usually, I'd take this as a sign to fuck off, but something made me wander over and ask him to repeat what he'd said.

'Those boots,' he said. 'They'll be no good if you aren't looking after your feet.'

'How do you mean?' I asked.

'I used to be in the navy,' he said. 'We used to have to run twenty miles with backpacks the size of yours and, if you didn't look after your feet, you'd end up with rancid toes.'

'What do you suggest?' I said. To my surprise, he handed me the spliff.

'Talc,' he said. 'At the start and end of every day. And if you get a minute to sit down occasionally, which I imagine you do' – he was army all right – 'then you need to take your shoes *and* socks off and let them breathe. Keeping your feet dry should be the thing you think about most if you're walking as far as you are . . . I'm assuming you're doing the coastal path?'

His appearance suggested he might be a little unhinged, but he was surprisingly sharp. I decided to tell him my route. The second I began to feel high, I was telling him everything, how I'd been dealing with suicidal thoughts and how I'd managed to rediscover a sense of purpose by setting myself this challenge. I found myself tailoring my story to suit him, emphasizing certain points as a way to connect as we passed the spliff back and forth. He listened intently, and once I'd finished he said:

'I've got some talc you can have back at mine. Follow me.'

He stood up, polished off his can with four or five hefty glugs, burped into his hand then beckoned me after him. I wasn't sure what to do. I had been perfectly happy sitting and shooting the breeze with this man, but did I really want to go back to his place? The weed that had facilitated a pleasant bonding experience was now making me slightly paranoid, and I was worried that if I said the wrong thing he might kick off. I took small steps, wondering whether I was judging him unfairly. He turned around.

'You coming or what?'

'Yes, mate, sorry. Lead the way,' I said, on pure instinct. It really is amazing the things I agree to in order to avoid potential conflict.

'And you can forget about camping, you're staying with me tonight.'

Shit, I thought.

'OK!' I said.

I began thinking about an exit strategy. *I could just turn around and run in the opposite direction* . . .

'Do you live alone?' I asked casually, trying to gather more info.

'No, my wife'll be home too,' he said.

'She doesn't know me, though, mate,' I said. 'Maybe we shouldn't just turn up? I'm fine camping, honestly,' I added desperately.

'Don't be daft. You're coming back, and that's the end of it. If she doesn't like it, that's her problem.'

I wracked my brain but I couldn't think of a good enough reason to say no, so on we walked. This will sound harsh, but I kind of expected to walk into a place that had the same vibe as the caravan I found myself in in Coverack – that appalling dog-hair and cigarette-smoke smell, shit everywhere, half a glass of unidentifiable brown liquid on the table. However, the house that the man led me to was anything but. It wasn't a grand house, by any stretch, but it was lovely, and when he opened the door and I peered inside it looked so clean and homely I genuinely thought that, despite him having a key, it might not be his house.

'Shoes off, please,' he said after we crossed the threshold. It smelt like lavender and fresh laundry; it was the nicest house I'd been in in weeks. I was halfway through taking off my boot when the man's wife, who must have heard us come in, appeared from a room at the end of the hall. She appeared, on first glance, very straight-laced, very professional. She had what I would describe as a 'corporate' hairstyle and was wearing a suit and smart shoes. You wouldn't have put them together in a million years. She approached with caution, and didn't take her eyes off me, staring me down like I was a bug in her tea.

'Who's this?' she said curtly, although her tone was more along the lines of 'Who *the fuck* is this?' I realized that, having judged the man I was with, I was now being judged, and considering I hadn't showered in about a week and was carrying a huge bag (which probably looked like it contained everything I possessed), I sensed I wasn't coming across too well. I also realized that the man and I were both really high and that he probably stank of beer. He couldn't have sold the idea of me staying any worse. And being high wasn't helping me.

'This is Jake. I just met him up the bus stop – he's gonna stay in the spare room.'

Her face turned stern. 'Can I talk to you for a minute?' she said to him.

The man looked at me and rolled his eyes.

Oh my god. Please don't do that, mate.

'Go and grab a shower, Jake, then come through to the kitchen when you're done,' he said.

As I removed my second boot a huge chunk of dry mud fell on to the clean carpet. I looked up. The woman's rage appeared to be boiling over, and through sheer awkwardness I made a beeline to what looked like the toilet door, which was open, without retrieving any soap or a towel from my bag. I brushed past the woman, let out an indecipherable sound that was probably a mixture of 'thank you' and 'sorry', got into the bathroom and shut myself inside. I heard the woman burst the second I locked the door.

'What the *fuck*, John?!'

'What?!'

'What are you playing at, inviting some vagrant into our house? What if he robs us in the night?!'

Fair point. But I was sure that John had my back and would reassure her that I was OK.

'If he robs us, I'll find him and I'll break his fucking legs!'

Maybe not.

I couldn't handle it. I stood in the bathroom, frozen and fully clothed, high as a kite, listening to two strangers argue *so* loudly about me. It was intense. Like being at a schoolfriend's house when their parents start rowing. Eventually, I decided that I was safe in the bathroom and that while I was there I might as well grab a shower. I'd only had the sea and a flannel to wash with for almost two months; the only showers I'd taken were when people had offered me a place to crash. I took off my clothes, stepped into the shower and spent the five or so minutes I was in there rehearsing what I was going to say to these people when the three of us were reunited. It was something along the lines of 'Look, you're clearly not comfortable with me being here, and I completely understand. I was going to camp anyway, so I'll just leave – I just wanted to say thanks for the shower.' A textbook charm offensive.

I winced when I realized I'd have to use one of their freshly washed towels and that I'd used their fancy soap. I dried myself off, put my dirty clothes back on and, very slowly, opened the door and walked to the kitchen. The door was shut, and I knocked, ever so gingerly.

'Come in!' a sprightly voice called out.

Not what I was expecting. I opened the door. In the kitchen, busying herself with various ingredients, was the woman.

'We were thinking of doing chicken, Jake. You're not vegetarian, are you?'

'Uh, yes. I mean no. I mean, I used to be but I'm not . . . chicken sounds lovely,' I said.

She was being too nice too soon after being so irate and it creeped me out. I looked across the room and saw John sitting at the dining table with two fresh cans of Tribute. As my eyes met his he slid one across the table and beckoned me to join him. For a second I felt like I might die in this house.

'Tell us all about your walk, Jake. It sounds fascinating,' said the woman.

It was surreal. All of a sudden, everything was completely cool, but instead of feeling relieved I was nervy. It didn't seem to make any sense.

What happened over the next few hours was unexpected – from feeling like I was intruding in the lives of two strangers, the three of us spent the evening in deep conversation about mostly very meaningful topics. John had indeed served in the military, and from what limited knowledge I have of post-traumatic stress, was perhaps experiencing some residual effects from that time. After a frosty start, the bulk of the evening's conversation was between me and John's wife, Pam; whenever John wanted to make a contribution he held his hand up until she noticed and kind of gave him permission to weigh in. They were an odd match but, despite their eccentricities, there was something about them that worked. They seemed quite comfortable in their roles, and by the time it was time to turn in I'd grown very fond of them. At one point of the evening, John asked, quite unexpectedly, if I liked 'art'.

'Well, sure . . .' I said.

'Show Jake your new painting,' John said to Pam excitedly.

Pam ushered me into the spare room, dug frantically around in the corner and pulled out a small canvas print. It was one of those cheap, tacky things you can buy from local markets and on it was a still from a Donald Duck film. I honestly thought it was a little joke the two of them had planned while I was in the shower, but when I looked at Pam, ready to laugh with her, it was clear she wanted my genuine opinion on it.

'Oh,' I said. 'Donald Duck.'

'Do you like Donald Duck?'

Mate.

'Yeah, well, I suppose you sort of have to, don't you?' I clutched.

'We *really* like Donald Duck,' said Pam.

'Oh . . . It's very nice.'

I bedded down that night in the room with the Donald Duck canvas propped against the wall, and after a quick look back over the evening, I chuckled myself to sleep.

The next day, I continued my journey along the SWCP, taking in the rugged precipices at Bedruthan Steps, where the rocks turned black and the waves beat the base of the cliffs mercilessly. A couple of days later I passed the white lighthouse at Hartland Point and entered the harbour village of Clovelly. My time in Cornwall had come to an end. It had taken me exactly a month to complete the four hundred-miles of Cornish coast, and as I crossed the border back into Devon I felt sad to be leaving.

Writing this now, I find myself contemplating why it felt so melancholic. I suppose it mostly boils down to feeling connected to Cornwall's kind, welcoming, often eccentric inhabitants. Humans are social animals and, despite the questionable gift of a leap in intelligence our species has been handed, we have to stay grounded enough to acknowledge our primal need for interaction. I lost sight of these things, which my mind and body craved, when I got sick, and it wasn't until the connections I made in Cornwall that I began to feel truly like I was part of the fabric of society again, and nothing, not walking or nature or talking about my feelings, has been half as effective for my mental health as feeling like I belong.

As sad as I was to be leaving Cornwall, it was exciting to be re-entering Devon. I decided that once I arrived at Exmoor National Park I'd give myself a break from the sea and head towards Minehead via the Coleridge Way. Some weeks previously in Dorset I had missed an opportunity to read the work of Thomas Hardy as I traversed the Hardy Way, so I decided to pick up a book of Coleridge's poems inspired by the area I was about to walk through. After three or four hours I came across a wide stream in the woods with stones big enough to sit on and decided there was the spot to sit and read some bloody poetry. I felt so scholarly, so educated . . . right up until I opened the book and read the opening line of the first poem. I didn't stay on that rock for long, and after realizing I was nowhere near clever enough to understand it, I honestly don't think I gave Coleridge's work another glance the whole time I was away. Even so, the decision to buy the book was encouraging and I took it as a sign that I was enjoying life again. The whole time I was working and living at the Well and Bucket I'd never picked up a book, never had any interest in learning anything new or gaining any type of new experience; all I could think to do to decompress was drink.

Using alcohol as a coping mechanism when you're seriously depressed is like putting a plaster over cancer. The occasional drink (or even big session) isn't inherently a bad thing, but when it becomes the only thing you're interested in and you start depriving yourself of things that *actually* make you feel better and replace them with mind-altering substances, you're on an express train to bigger, scarier, more personalized issues. It feels trite to describe it as a slippery slope, but that's exactly what it is.

After my failed attempt at being highbrow, I stuffed my newly acquired book of indecipherable poetry to the bottom of my pack and continued west through the crisp woods and fields of Exmoor. It wouldn't be long before I reached Minehead, and as I neared the end point of the South West Coast Path I was hit by a sudden, unexpected wave of anxiety after packing the Flea down one morning a few miles west of Porlock. The cause of the knot in my stomach wasn't immediately clear, but I knew it had something to do with my uncertainty about the road ahead. The South West Coast Path had been a reliable place of safety for me over the past six weeks – hugging the coastlines of Dorset, Devon and Cornwall had, of course, been exhausting at times, but with the sea always to my left it had been relatively easy to keep my bearings and stay on track. For some reason, though, immersed in the thick green of Exmoor, I felt conflicted. I was excited by the prospect of completing one of Great Britain's longest and most scenic trails but at the same time perturbed by the reality of what I would (literally) be walking into next.

After Minehead, I was to carry on along the coast to Portishead, then Bristol, then into a whole other country – Wales. I was thinking about how the ocean wouldn't be in sight again until I reached the Pembrokeshire coast, and the thought of hiking inland trails in an unfamiliar and far less populated part of the UK was filling me with an unexpected nervousness.

I reminded myself how far I'd come and how strong I felt physically. My legs had proved themselves up to the task by carrying me almost eight hundred miles across England in two months. I felt motivated, confident and was thinking more clearly than I had in a very, very long time, but in that moment my mind struggled to withstand a thundering reality check.

In the end I decided I was just going to try and enjoy this last little bit of Exmoor. The scenery was breathtaking – your archetypal English countryside, complete with oak trees, sheep and the occasional scattering of colour from various wild flowers. It was the perfect time of year to be exploring such a romantic part of England and I found that the more I focused on my surroundings, the less I agonized about the future.

It felt like I'd needed that little change of scenery, like

breaking up the six hundred-plus miles of coast I'd traversed had allowed me to take stock and think about my journey in a more realistic way.

The final miles between Porlock and Minehead felt like a dream, and as I scaled the narrow footpath around the edge of Selworthy Beacon I stopped to admire the view. Waves crashed dramatically into the bases of coarse, angular cliffs and the bright green grass and pink and yellow heather that cloaked the clifftops rolled into the distance as far as I could see. I became so lit up with energy that I almost felt like running the last few miles. When I could see Minehead under a mile or so away, I turned to take one last look at the coastal path. It had been six weeks since I had stepped off the toll ferry in Poole and taken my first steps on the beach at Studland Peninsula and, despite everything that had happened since then, all the people I'd met and connected with so deeply, every beach and town and weird situation I'd found myself in that at the time I was sure I'd remember forever, in the moment I crossed the marker in Minehead I could barely remember any of it. All I knew was that I felt I had accomplished something massive and I felt proud and slightly amazed at how far I'd come.

It was now approaching September, almost half a year to the day since I'd been a moment from ending my life, and now here I was, living it better than I ever knew was possible. I thought about the contrast between how I felt in March and the way I felt here, now, how sure I had been that I would never see this motivated, adventurous side of me again.

Over the following week I traipsed the sixty or so miles to Portishead via the Somerset coast path, ducking inland only to cross the rivers through Bridgwater and Burnham-on-Sea, and again to get from Brean to Weston-super-Mare.

Time moved very quickly. I spent a lot of it reflecting on my life, remembering how little I had wanted it just half a year previously, and realizing how much I valued it now. My body was tired, but it didn't matter. It was keeping my mental strength up that was going to prove most important in completing my challenge – staying disciplined when the road got hard, staying positive when my morale was low, and staying focused on the reasons why I was out there in the first place.

From Avonmouth I joined the Severn Way, passing through the Bristol suburbs, Severn Beach and Redwick as I edged closer and closer to the Welsh border. The banks of the Severn were a little rough-looking, a bit neglected and unloved. Maybe it was just the grey sky that had crept in as I edged towards the Severn Bridge that made the landscape appear so bleak, but there was so much industry in the surrounding area my sense of awe, which had been so present in recent weeks, felt distinctly lacking. For some reason, I'd romanticized the Severn Bridge, envisaging a sort of cobbled canal-type viaduct that had stood strong in Welsh rock for centuries. In reality, the road into Wales appeared to be just a busy 5,000-yard motorway suspension bridge.

As I got closer I realized I'd finally reached a point in my journey where I was afraid to walk the road ahead of me. I hadn't been waiting for it, but now it was here I was surprised it had taken as long as it had. I really didn't want to set foot on that bridge. It looked like death. It was so long, and there were so many cars tearing up and down the six lanes. Having no other play available to me, I carried on walking towards it, hoping some sort of solution would present itself. Now, I could see a few workmen in hi-vis jackets looking perfectly relaxed and safe on the bridge about fifty yards ahead of me. To my relief, on the far-left-hand side of the road was a walkway that ran the length of the entire bridge.

The wind had picked up and was blowing the rain sideways into my face, but as I began to cross the bridge I was struck by how little I cared about the weather. It didn't matter. I had walked the length of the country and was about to enter Wales. It had been eighty-two days and around eight hundred miles since I'd left Brighton, which I know, speed-wise, doesn't exactly make me Haile Gebrselassie, but it was by far the greatest achievement of my life. In fact, I was beginning to see every new mile as a new greatest achievement of my life. Tomorrow would be my life's greatest achievement, and the following day, and so on. Regardless of how many miles I was averaging per day, I was winning, and after feeling like a loser for so much of my life I allowed myself to feel proud of what I had accomplished.

9

My excitement at walking into another country was sweet but short-lived. As the Severn Bridge led me over the final sliver of English land, Beachley Point, the dark clouds that had been slowly forming throughout the day split and drenched me the minute I set foot in Wales. Classic. After a blazing summer, I was beginning to think that the next few months would present a different, wetter, set of inconveniences. Thankfully, however, that afternoon I had plans that couldn't be ruined by rain. I'd been invited to the Mental Health Foundation's Cardiff office to chat to the staff.

I'd chosen to raise money for the MHF completely randomly. I wasn't familiar with any mental health charities before I began my walk, and I ended up spending all of about four minutes scrolling through Google search results before concluding that they all do important work and that I should just pick one. It worked out perfectly in the end, as the MHF have three offices – one in Cardiff, one in Edinburgh and one in London – one for each country I'd be passing through on my route around Britain. When I arrived in the Welsh capital after a short train ride from Chepstow I was greeted with tea, Jaffa Cakes and huge smiles from the team, just what I fancied after being soaked to my mantle.

Mental health charities are hugely important, as they attempt to scoop up those who are failed by other mental health systems that, sadly, are stretched unbelievably thin as they are. The MHF offers information to those in need of some understanding of mental-health issues and promotes effective self-management tools and preventative measures to promote a more healthy mental well-being. As I was briefed on the team's objectives I remember thinking how helpful their service might have been to me while I was in crisis. They provide a much-needed ear to really listen to people in need of help, and I felt sure I'd made a good decision to try and help their cause through my challenge.

Despite tactically choosing a chair next to a radiator and spending a few hours there, my clothes were still damp when I left the office, so I decided, as I was in the city, to loosen the purse strings and check myself into a hostel. The days were getting noticeably shorter and conditions were on the turn. The days it didn't stop raining at all were the worst. Walking all day, getting soaked and attempting to pitch the Flea and get in it without getting the inside wet seemed virtually impossible, but it got easier with practice. The trick, I found, was to set the tent up as swiftly as possible, leave my towel in the porch area, strip every item of clothing off and 'Superman' into the tent the second I'd given myself a onceover. The towel is the vital component, obviously, so if you're thinking of adopting this technique, you must be sure that you apply due diligence in retrieving your towel from your bag the following day and, if you're treated to dry weather or even a ray of sun, hang it on your pack to dry it off, ready to repeat the process that evening, if that's what the weather dictates. The things that, unfortunately, can't be sorted out and you just have to get over (if you're planning on walking for weeks and months on end like me, that is) are putting cold, wet clothes back on the following day (they will have got absolutely freezing in the night, by the way) and rolling up a wet tent if it's still drizzly the next morning. The smell of damp and mould would become a part of me as I traipsed around Wales, an annoyingly predictable feature of an otherwise beautiful country.

Once I'd got the train back to Chepstow, I began heading north to Monmouth, sixteen miles away. I'd arranged to stay with my aunt Debby there during my first couple of days in Wales. It was a little out of the way but still a worthwhile walk along the Wye Valley, which is largely made up of dense woodland so, for the most part, offered some shelter from the weather. The two days I stayed with Debs was probably the most time I'd ever spent with her. She's the daughter of my step-grandad, Norman, and while I have hazy memories of playing with her in Nan and Norm's garden, she didn't feature very heavily in my childhood. That said, while we never spent enough time around each other to really get close, I was always fond of Debs. She always had this little smirk on her face, like she always had a private running joke in her head. It felt great to finally get to know her and establish a more adult relationship; it felt that by doing so I was strengthening the ties to my more distant family, something I never really considered might be a nice thing to do before.

I also spent my time there preparing to take on national park number four, the Brecon Beacons. I felt so much better knowing I was heading into the mountains with clean pants and socks and a dry tent I could breathe in without the risk of inhaling mould spores.

After saying goodbye to Auntie Debs I headed west, towards the mountains, smelling like shampoo and fabric softener. It took a couple of days to get to Brecon via the Monmouthshire and Brecon canal, a winding but very flat pathway that reminded me of the canal path that joins my home town of Maldon to Heybridge Basin. I must have been tuned into the thought of home after spending time with my aunt. As I plodded through various locks and neighbouring villages, I thought about the length of my journey and how long it might be before I would see my friends and family again, and before I smelt the distinctive wooden smell of Mum's boat.

Around this time I received an unexpected message from an old friend from back home who I hadn't spoken to in about ten years. It wasn't that uncommon for old friends to suddenly make contact since I began the walk, but Fia's message was different to many of the messages I'd receive. She told me that a friend of hers who worked in TV was putting together a project and she thought I'd be good for it. She didn't know much about it, other than it would be a TV programme about mental health, but she offered to put my name forward. I expressed as much confused interest as I could muster, before she asked me: 'Have you ever run a marathon?'

I replied no, and that was that.

I arrived in Brecon three days and thirty-five miles later, and the first order of business was to find an outdoor recreation store. After three months of setting it up and taking it down virtually every day, the Flea was in need of some minor repairs. He had served me incredibly well up to that point, but his poles had started to warp and his zips were getting stiff and, although there were no discernible holes or tears, in a few patches he was beginning to look worn. I felt that a quick service from someone who knows about tents might get me through the next few months before I had to think about buying a replacement.

I found a camping store and, within thirty seconds of spotting me, the sales guy was on me like a bumblebee on a lavender bush. He must have taken me as a serious outdoors-man and, much like when I worked in a music shop when I was eighteen, the ability to tell apart the veterans and the rookies who wander into your shop becomes a bit of a skill, and a good way of deciding who or who not to devote your time trying to sell things to. At this stage, having covered a distance of almost a thousand miles, I think I had, to that guy at least, the look of a hiking veteran, which was actually a nice change to people in supermarkets staring dubiously at me like I was just a man who might live in the woods.

'Blimey, where have you come from?' he said, struggling to curb his enthusiasm as he looked me up and down. He had a pierced eyebrow and about twenty leather bracelets, and was countering the fact that he was going bald *and* grey with black hair dye and a very carefully thought-out hairstyle.

'I've, well, I've walked here from Brighton,' I said shyly. Something about telling people this was beginning to feel weird – like it was too long a distance to be real. I could tell that this guy believed me, though, or wanted to believe me, at least.

'Wow.' There was an awkward pause as he appeared to briefly forget his role in the customer – shop assistant dynamic. 'Oh, is there something I can help you with today?' he added, remembering.

I voiced my concerns about my tent and asked if the store provided some sort of repair service.

'What model is it you have?' he asked.

'It's a Wild Country Zephyros 2,' I said, catching myself before referring to it as 'Flea'.

'Hold on just a moment,' he said, and zipped excitedly towards the back of the shop and through a 'Staff Only' door. He returned a few moments later, wide-eyed, carrying what appeared to be another Zephyros 2, with no mud or leaves or grass stains on it.

'This was a display model we got sent a few months back and never got round to using,' he said. 'You can have it!'

'I can ... have it?' I echoed hesitantly, unsure that I'd understood correctly.

He thrust the tent into my arms then stepped back, holding his hands up to indicate that he was absolutely sure.

This gesture, as well as the overall level of kindness that had been coming my way over the past few months, was astounding. Everywhere I went people insisted on offering me things – a lift, a place to stay, a meal here, a new tent there ... I felt indebted to everyone who had helped me. None of them had asked for anything in return, which often left me feeling a bit befuddled, like staring at a sum that didn't add up. *People are always after something, no matter how kind they're coming off* chimed an internal voice that sounded suspiciously like my old man's. But the more I recalled those acts of kindness, the more I could see that people were just helping because they wanted to, because they believed in something about what I was doing. Although I had become aware of the respect people had for me taking on this challenge some time ago, I now saw that what I was doing really meant something to them. The fact that I was doing it all in the name of mental health seemed to be reaching them on an emotional level. It was a huge realization, one that made me consider afresh the idea that maybe this walk and what it represented was bigger than me, that the downfall that had ultimately facilitated it was also the key to unlocking some kind of potential in other people, as well as my own.

With a fresh new tent and a feeling like I was existing in the greatest time of my life, I left the shop and began heading south, into the mountains.

The Brecon Beacons are mostly covered in vast green blankets, making them appear more like hills from a distance. In the very centre sits Pen y Fan, the highest peak in South

Wales, at 886 metres above sea level. It's an amazing experience, walking to the top of a mountain. It's a challenge I would recommend to anyone – the sense of achievement of standing atop a mountain you've just scaled is so unique, so empowering, and looking out for miles is a profoundly moving experience. The summit of Pen y Fan joins on to the summit of another mountain, Corn Du, which is smaller but equally as pretty as her neighbour. The trail that spans the length of these two mountains is well visited and was pleasantly easy to navigate.

When I reached the bottom I began to scout out a place to camp. My legs were starting to seize up and I'd been experiencing some discomfort on my left side; it was the first thing I'd encountered that I could confidently call a 'niggle' – not bad going, I suppose, considering it was the first I'd had in about nine hundred miles, but it felt like something to keep an eye on.

I set my new tent up at the base of Corn Du before it got dark so I could get an early night and rest up, but I couldn't get into bed until maybe an hour or so later, because the second I unzipped the door a massive toad jumped inside it. I panicked and zipped it inside and watched it freak out and bounce around like a pinball until it tired itself out and I got enough confidence to open the zip and give it its chance to escape. It was easily the most stressful part of the walk to date. I christened my new tent 'the Toad'.

The Beacons Way trail took me over one final summit, Fan Llia, before spitting me out into the Swansea Valley. After a week's worth of natural Welsh splendour I was about to re-enter civilization.

Camping in cities is a big no-no. The parks might look safe enough during the day, but that can all change when the sun goes down. Day folk are replaced by night folk, buggies by druggies. It doesn't always kick off, but if you're camping in a city park you'll likely spend your whole night worrying it might. Saying that, Swansea's a nice city. The bustle in the centre felt energizing rather than aggressive, and at just eleven miles away from the first AONB I'd visit, the Gower Peninsula, the sandy coastline that cradles the city's south side makes for a very appealing setting. It was so scenic that I thought about camping right on the beach when I first arrived, but reasoned that if there's a no parks rule, there would probably be a no city beaches rule too.

It was getting late, though – the walk through the Swansea Valley from Ystradgynlais had taken longer than planned – so when I arrived at the coast by Swansea University it was already dark and I had no plan. I'd seen on the map that there was what I had got used to referring to as a 'patch of green', but after checking it out it still felt too close to the city centre and simply not safe enough to pitch a tent in. I checked the prices of a few hotels and B&Bs, but they were all too pricey or too full. I was in a pickle, a potentially serious one.

I wandered back into the city centre, which was, thankfully, not too rowdy, to grab something to eat and come up with a plan. After a decadent city meal of Chicken McNuggets and fries, I decided that my best course of action would be to go to a pub and get chatting to someone long enough for them to let me crash at their place. Absolute nightmare of a plan, but it was either that or chance it in the woods and risk getting my tent sicked on by a young, drunk chav. I had a quick google for any local rock or metal bars, and found two. In Bristol I'd ended up at a grotty metal dive (in the nicest possible sense) and was offered a couch to crash on upwards of twenty times by four or five different bearded chaps wearing either Iron Maiden, Meshuggah or Lamb of God T-shirts. Folks in the metal community are often some of the loveliest people you'll ever meet, so I picked the better reviewed of the two pubs and walked there. I had enough cash on me for a few pints and, with a charm offensive and the right balance of self-assuredness, humbleness and knowledge of one or two math-metal bands, I was fairly confident I'd be tucked up on a grotty sofa beneath a System of a Down poster by midnight.

As I approached I heard the unmistakable sound of AC/DC filter into the street. This was definitely the right place. Pushing the door open, I was hit with the classic metal bar stench of sweaty men and unwashed beer lines. I strolled over to the bar and, in a vague attempt to attract some attention, air-drummed along to a few bars of 'Thunderstruck' while I waited to get served. Standing at the bar next to me were a couple of textbook greebos (as was the expression back in school). I immediately began to feel like this plan was a lot more doable in my head and that striking up a conversation with a stranger in the hope they might ask if I wanted to stay at their house was actually unbelievably awkward and a bit creepy. Thankfully, one of the two gentlemen had already clocked my pack, which I'd wedged between two bar stools strategically in plain view, so I hoped all I had to do for him to start talking to me was maybe meet his gaze briefly once or twice and strike the second their conversation petered out.

In the end, all it took was for me to ask them to watch my bag while I went to the loo and thanking them when I got back. I banked on their curiosity being what provoked an actual conversation and, mercifully, I was right. Within five minutes they had bought me a pint and were staring at me, as most people tended to, with wide, inquisitive eyes, excitedly asking me all about my journey. Their names were Gaz and Jamie, and they were both local. Gaz was the quieter of the two – a big guy with a small presence, a slightly nervous smile, short, thinning dark hair and the inability to look anyone, it would seem, in the eye for longer than a second. He wore a black-and-red chequered shirt, an old pair of jeans that had completely lost their fit and an even older pair of – I guess – green DC skate shoes. He basically looked like every bloke in every metal bar in every country in the Western world.

Jamie was of average height and stocky and held himself with an unapologetic confidence that I was immediately drawn to. He had the air of a roadie – the energetic bloke who tours with the band, sets up the drums, drinks fifteen beers and makes jokes that he always finds funnier than the person he's telling them to; basically, the sort of guy everyone loves. He had a grown-out mohawk and his clothes were faded black and slightly damp with sweat. Again, exactly the type of guy you'd expect to find in that sort of place. Jamie and I bonded quickly – he seemed like a genuine and decent lad – and after about half an hour of discussing my walk and the various bands we both like, the two of us went outside for a smoke. The night air was bitterly cold, and the smoke from our cigarettes, infused with the air evaporating from our mouths, bellowed into thick clouds that hung all around us. In a moment of silence, without thinking too much about it, I decided to just go for it.

'Jamie, I'm sorry to ask this, but I'm in a real jam. I've got nowhere to stay tonight . . . Is there any chance I can crash on your sofa?'

Jamie looked back at me without expression, the remnants of his last puff slowly cascading from his nostrils before disappearing into the night. It was the first time I'd asked for a place to stay rather than being offered one, and I immediately recognized the (quite colossal) difference between the two. I waited self-consciously as Jamie's stare lingered, weighing it up. He looked torn, like he would normally say yes to someone who asked but had decided, on this occasion, to really mull it over. After a few seconds he held up his hand, the palm facing me and fingers splayed, and took a short breath before he said:

'OK, look, Jake. You seem cool, but let's hang out here for a bit first, have a few more beers and I'll decide in a bit?'

'Of course,' I said, and with that we both nodded awkwardly, stubbed out our cigarettes and headed inside. He could not have responded more fairly, and I respected him for not just saying yes before properly sizing up the favour. Twenty minutes later it all came together as Jamie suggested the three of us stop spending all our money in the pub, grab some cans and head over to his place. The relief washed over me like a cool shower and I hastily polished off the last of my pint and got ready to go.

On the way, Jamie insisted we walk a slightly longer way so he could show me a tunnel that had, as he described it, 'perfect reverb'. Jamie was a real sound junkie; he'd studied music production at uni and had been DJing around shift work at the bar where he worked full time since then. He lived alone, and it looked like it. His sofa faced an obscenely large TV that was mounted on the wall and between them sat a coffee table that bore a striking resemblance to the coffee tables of my old house shares in Brighton, complete with overflowing ashtrays, empty beer cans, Xbox controllers, all peppered with a good pinch of dry tobacco. The walls had probably been white once but were now stained yellow and featured no sort of decoration except, to my delight, a slightly creased System of a Down poster.

Gaz and I sat down while Jamie nipped to the kitchen to

'grab something'. He returned with three cans, a little wooden smoking box and a bag of speed. Needless to say, over the following five or six hours the evening shifted through several new gears – the initial jump to lightspeed lasted maybe an hour before the pace began to drop, then the ability to form coherent sentences abandoned us all, one by one. Gaz tapped out and was out of the door by 2 a.m., leaving Jamie and me to pontificate well into the daylight hours.

It's a situation that I, to my shame, was still catching myself falling into all too easily. When drugs are just a normal part of life, it gets really easy to just say yes to them; even if you know it's going to be rubbish the following day or, if you're like me, the following week. If you're reading this and thinking that it doesn't really sound worth it, you'd be absolutely right. But. That logic simply doesn't seem to compute sometimes, especially when drugs are introduced after booze, resulting in evenings like the one I spent with Jamie, where hanging out stopped being fun at some point and turned into a shouting match where the choice phrase became: 'The thing about me is, right . . .'

That's not to say I didn't enjoy my night at Jamie's, or Jamie himself. He was a great host and we had very natural chemistry. When he finally called it a night at around 8 a.m., saying goodnight to him felt like saying goodnight to an old friend.

I woke the next day to the sound of Jamie bundling down the stairs. It was 2.30 p.m. *Shit. He's going to kick me out. He's going to kick me out and I feel like I've had no sleep and I'm going to have to walk miles today on a comedown. Fuck! This is Adam's all over again.*

I sat up sluggishly.

'Morning.'

'Morning.'

It was a little awkward. I'd met Jamie after he'd already had a skinful in the pub, and by the time we'd piled back to his he was completely cooked. Now here we were, face to face in the cold light of day, me feeling like I'd slightly duped him into staying with him, him realizing he'd let a total stranger crash on his sofa, and both of us on what I assumed was an equally crushing comedown. As horrendous as I felt, I decided the right thing to do was leave.

'Thanks so much for letting me stay, man. Gimme twenty minutes and I'll be out of your hair,' I said.

Jamie looked at me through expressionless glassy eyes. He looked like he was going to throw up right there.

'No way, man,' he eventually said, his voice much deeper than it had been the night before. 'You look like how I feel right now. I've got work in an hour, but you chill here as long as you want, order in food, stay another night – whatever. I'll be back around midnight.'

I didn't know what to say. I couldn't believe it. After some light conversation over a coffee, Jamie set the TV up for me, showed me how it all worked then left, leaving me in absolutely the best environment to deal with the mistakes (drugs) I made (took) the night before – on my own, in a warm house.

People find it strange when I say I like my own company, considering how low I can get sometimes. The reason is that I like being around people but I also find it a lot of work. I heard the term 'extroverted introvert' once and, despite not being one for pigeonholing myself, I do kind of identify with it. It's important to be social, even when the idea of being around people is a bit much sometimes. The feeling of being alone and detached from society is a powerful one, and in my experience people who cut themselves off from others tend to get a bit bitter, resentful and weird around people, and just a bit angry at the world. It's not how I want to live, so although I do indulge in alone time more than a lot of my friends do, I also try to balance that out with quality time with people I like, and most of the time that's fine for me. During the walk I was able to instil this more or less to perfection, by walking alone all day, with folks breezing in and out of my life. That's why when Jamie not only said I could chill at his that day but that he was going *out*, I may as well have won the lottery.

I nodded off peacefully for another hour or so. When I awoke, I showered, ordered a takeaway and proceeded to play FIFA on Jamie's massive telly until I crashed out at about 10 p.m.

It had been months since I'd had the pleasure of home comforts, and after a good ten-hour slumber I felt refreshed and ready to carry on heading west towards the Pembroke-shire coast. I'd missed Jamie getting in the night before and had woken up before him that day. When he surfaced at around 10 a.m., I was packed up and ready to leave.

'Morning.'

'Morning.'

Much more relaxed this time. In fact, I was really pleased to see Jamie. He looked rested, and pleased to see me too.

'I'm all packed up, mate, I just wanted to say thanks again in person before I left,' I said.

Jamie stared at me for a second, a look of disappointment etched on to his face.

'All right, that's cool,' he said. 'I was going to suggest that we maybe do something today. You've been here two days and you haven't seen Swansea at all.'

He went on to suggest a load of cool things – get lunch at the market, see the buildings that were bombed during the

Swansea Blitz, get a drink at the top of a high-rise building with a view over the city . . . it felt like he'd planned a whole day for us, and I realized this was a rare opportunity to get to know a place I was passing through. With that, I left my pack where it was and after a quick coffee the two of us headed out. We did everything Jamie had listed – we got Thai food from the market, Jamie flexed his impressive knowledge about which buildings were destroyed in the German bombings of 1941 and, finally, the two of us scaled the Meridian Tower and cheersed our day out with a cold beer as we gazed out over the city.

I'd met a lot of people since 27 June, when I left Brighton, but no one had gone to as much effort as Jamie. He made me realize how much I missed my friends, and whereas, before, I'd given myself a hard time for indulging in these types of destructive behaviours, I wasn't consumed with regret on this occasion. It felt worth it. Jamie was a good bloke, but at the same time I couldn't shake the feeling that there was something else going on, something driving his kindness. After we finished our beers the two of us went back to his house, and that's when it all came out.

A couple of months previously, Jamie had fallen victim to a home invasion. He'd been chilling in his living room one evening when three men burst into his house, stole all of his high-priced possessions, and bundled Jamie into the back of a van at knife point. Jamie was, thankfully, able to give his captors the slip before the van drove away, and escaped on foot. He informed the police, who caught the three men later that day. Jamie said he recognized one of the invaders, which not only made it easier for the police to track him down but also for Jamie to speculate on what had happened. The person he recognized was an associate of some, as Jamie put it, 'dodgy cunts'. Jamie reasoned that this guy – all three of them, perhaps – was in debt to someone quite scary, and that by robbing Jamie, selling all his electronic goods and intimidating him into clearing his bank account out, they'd be able to clear their debt.

This is all conjecture, of course, but it seemed to make sense how Jamie told it. The thing I couldn't get my head around was how he could allow me, a complete stranger, to crash with him, in the same house, so soon after something so traumatizing occurred there. When I said this to him, I was humbled when he responded by telling me that I was 'clearly a good guy'; he said that 'one incident shouldn't stop me from letting good people into my life'.

I was devastated for Jamie, of course I was. He didn't deserve that. But I sensed that something about what had happened to him had helped him in some way. He appeared to have not only made his peace with it but had used his experience to strengthen his natural benevolence. He wasn't a slave to his trauma, he owned it, and that inspired me. It inspired me to try and appreciate something that I already felt like I was on the cusp of – reworking my memory of lying in bed in my room in Shoreditch, wanting to die, so that it had a purpose. I could even learn to be thankful for that day, because without it I'd never be doing what I was doing now. I might not have come to have the same amount of empathy for others who experience pain as I once did. Opening up had brought me closer to everybody around me, made me want to be egoless and stopped me questioning who I was better or worse off than. It had taught me to be kind, to think about *why* people act and not to be so quick to judge their actions.

I walked for four or five days before I spoke to Jamie again. In that time, a journalist friend of mine who was working for *Men's Health* had been in touch to ask if I could make a video about the walk for their website. They needed it in a specific file format that I couldn't do on my phone, so without anyone else I could really ask, I called Jamie to see if he could help. He told me to jump on a train and head back to Swansea the next day, that he was at work but would leave a key under the mat, and that he'd help me with it when he got home. I arrived at his place around 5 p.m. I went in, let my bag drop to the floor and was about to go to the toilet when I noticed, next to an unopened can of lager, a small chalkboard that had been positioned upright on the kitchen counter, facing the door. On it, Jamie had written, 'Welcome home, bruv.'

Wales was the first country in the world to have a pathway that spans the entire coastline. For some reason, the Wales Coast Path isn't registered as a national trail, but at a hefty 870 miles it eclipses the length of the South West Coast Path (the 'official' longest trail in Britain) by almost 250 miles. It begins (or ends, depending on which way you do it) in Chepstow, the first town I entered after crossing the Severn Bridge, but as I'd decided to take a small detour through the Brecon Beacons my journey along the Welsh coast officially began at the Gower Peninsula, one of the most beautiful sections of coast in the entire British Isles. Vast sand beaches emerge from behind a sea of dunes that disappear behind miles of rugged coastline. Despite the grey skies and cold Atlantic breeze that loomed over me as I continued west, the charm of the Gower, and the entire Welsh coast for that matter, was never lost on me.

I'd got as far as Carmarthen after leaving Jamie's, and after a quick hop back to Swansea so he could help me with the video, I returned to Wales's oldest town by train. It was a little disheartening, to be honest: it took forty minutes on a train, but it had taken me nearly a week on foot.

Things were beginning to annoy me – bad weather, sore feet, putting my tent up every day, putting my tent away every day, not knowing where I was half the time, having stones in my boots, the wind, having to shit outdoors in broad daylight, saying hello to someone and them not saying hello back . . . I'd been on the road for a hundred days and I suppose the novelty was beginning to wear off. The walking part of my day had become my equivalent of a working day, and my downtime was limited either to sitting alone in my tent with 4G, or sitting alone in my tent without 4G. I was getting irritable. I needed something exciting to happen – I needed some motivation.

I'd been following the progress of some 'adventure athletes' – other people who had embarked on out-sized endurance challenges. One guy called Sean Conway had completed a 4,000-mile ultra-triathlon around Britain, while Elise Downing and Simon Clark were running the entire British coastline. While Elise had already completed her lap of the UK by the time I reached Wales, Simon was still out there somewhere, living his challenge every day, as I was. I sometimes thought how cool it would be to run into him; he'd been traversing the British coast counter-clockwise, the opposite direction to me, which made the chances pretty good.

I'd left Jamie's at around five, so by the time I rolled into Carmarthen the darkness was setting in. There was a playing field next to the university on the outskirts of town that looked safe enough to camp in, or at least it did on the map, so I began walking straight there as soon as I got off the train. As I marched up the high street I noticed a man with long, fluffy white hair coming down it and recognized him immediately.

It was Simon Clark.

Simon's hair is kind of his trademark, but in case there was any confusion he also wore a bright-pink top underneath an ultra-running vest bearing the words: 'Run around Britain'. His features were delicate and birdlike and the tip of his nose glowed pink – a sure sign he'd been spending all his days outside. I approached him with shamelessly visible intent to get into his eyeline and, to my initial disappointment, he returned my gaze with a look that said, 'I really can't be arsed with you, mate.' I thought about leaving him alone for all of two seconds before deciding that the chance to meet someone else yomping around Britain was simply too rare to let go.

It didn't matter anyway, in the end, because as soon as I announced that I knew who he was I quickly found out that the initial cagey look he gave me was simply because people kept telling him he looked like Jimmy Savile, which I imagine wasn't that funny even the first time – even though he would probably admit that, due to his hair, he kind of did. Anyway, the second Simon realized I recognized him for who he was, his mood seemed to lift. When I told him I was also circumnavigating mainland Britain, his reaction almost made me cry. His blue eyes shimmered and he grabbed me by the shoulders, pulled me towards him and said, somewhat cryptically: 'I didn't realize you were a brother!'

We embraced for maybe five or six seconds longer than your average hug, and I felt the love that (I would eventually come to realize) constantly radiates out of Simon.

He was running around Britain to raise funds for Ecologia, a charity that works to support disadvantaged children and young people in Scotland, where Simon lives, as well as in Russia and several countries in Africa. He was running ten to twenty miles every day and sleeping in a bivvy bag every night, which, I remember thinking, was way more hardcore than what I was doing. After our truly excellent hug Simon told me he was looking for a place to eat before he bedded down for the night. I still needed to go and check out a place where I thought I could pitch the Toad, so we exchanged numbers and agreed to meet for breakfast somewhere in town the following day.

I found a decent enough spot to camp, and as I lay in my tent I thought about the relative luxury I was in compared to Simon, who was essentially sleeping in a body bag. I reasoned that feeling bad for him in any way was completely the wrong way of looking at it – he was on the adventure of his life, just like I was, and the discomfort and laborious nature of it was all part of it. Simon's life mirrored my own at that time, and our chance meeting couldn't have come at a better time for me. It made me realize just how lucky I was to be doing what I was doing and reminded me that, despite my recent dip in mood, this would likely be the most fulfilling time of my life, maybe even the only time I would be able to exist in this way. The walk didn't feel like a challenge anymore, it felt like a lifestyle, so I had to expect all the downs and upswings that went with that.

Simon and I met the following morning at a quiet café on Carmarthen High Street, as planned. We hung out for two hours or so, sharing stories from the road and telling each other what we could expect in the upcoming miles. Simon was heading south towards the South West Coast Path, while I was about to enter the Pembrokeshire Coastal Path. I would come to realize the two are hugely similar landscapes. When we finished eating we had yet another lingering and heartfelt embrace before setting off in opposite directions.

Watching him pick up his pace and disappear down the street, I wondered how different his experience had been to mine. It occurred to me that running every day instead of walking might not actually be that much tougher on a body physically, considering the extra hours of downtime he'd have. In fact, getting that mileage done in a faster time with nothing on your back might be easier in some ways. The more I pondered the idea of running, the more it excited me. Walking was great, but I felt determined and inspired by Simon. I fantasized about abandoning my pack, buying a pair of trail running shoes and running the whole 180 miles of the Pembrokeshire coast as a sort of challenge *within* a challenge. Funny how, no matter how fulfilled you are with your current life, there will always be someone to compare yourself to. There I was, on the adventure of a lifetime, and all it took was one conversation to make me wish I was more like someone else.

Obviously, deep down, I knew there was no way I could do what Simon was doing. I was in better shape than I'd been six months previously, granted, but I was nowhere near the level of fitness I needed to be to do what he was doing. I was still smoking, drinking, and occasionally taking drugs – it was actually pretty amazing I'd got as far as I had. But I was determined, and driven, and dogged. I felt like I was capable of a lot more than I'd previously have thought possible, and so when I received an email a few days after bumping into Simon asking if I'd be interested in running the London Marathon as part of an upcoming BBC documentary about mental health, I wasted no time in responding. Fia had obviously done what she said she was going to, and put my name forward. *Jesus – the London Marathon.*

Filming was due to begin in November, which meant that in order to take part I was going to have to do something unprecedented. I was going to have to put a pin in the walk. It was already October, and the days were getting colder. Some nights I'd wake up in the Toad shivering, and it was only going to get more intense over winter, especially once I got up to Scotland. The ache on my left side, which I'd done well to ignore, for the most part, was also getting harsher.

The more I thought about it, the more a winter break seemed like a sensible thing to do – with or without the documentary. It felt right to take a break, and after a few email exchanges I agreed, in principle, to take part in a project called 'Mind over Marathon' – a very snappy title, I remember thinking.

I had about a month and a half to walk as far as I could. I plotted a route and set myself a target of reaching Edale, in Derbyshire – the start point of the 268-mile Pennine Way, which runs north from central England into central Scotland. I thought that would be a suitable place to begin the second half of my walk. For the moment, however, I had to focus on the task in front of me, and after a few more emails I continued west on to the Pembrokeshire coast path. I spent the following days walking peacefully and excitedly through some of the most amazing stretches of coast, daydreaming about what it was going to be like to run the London Marathon. It was exciting, and I felt so lucky to be alive . . . right up until I reached Pembroke, where everything came crashing down.

Pembroke isn't technically on the coastal path, but to continue walking west in a way that was both time and effort efficient it made sense to cut through the town and cross the bridge over to Neyland before continuing on. It was dark by the time I got into Pembroke and, unexpectedly, the town was alive with bright lights, loud music and hordes of people eating hot dogs and candyfloss. I spotted a toffee-apple stall through the gauntlet of sparklers and mums in puffa coats and, from not having thought about toffee apples since I was a child, in that moment I wanted one more than I'd ever wanted anything else. I was conscious that me and my pack took up more than our fair share of room, so before I indulged I made my way over to a set of steps that led away from the high street, down towards a clearing that looked hidden enough for me to pitch my tent. My 'no parks' rule was hastily shoved to the back of my mind while the toffee apple took centre stage. The weariness of a long day was setting in and, coupled with a desire to absorb some of the buzz, I decided it would be safe enough to pitch near the crowds of families enjoying some good clean fun. If anything, in this scenario, the person sleeping in a tent in a city park would be the one to be avoided.

However, less than a minute after I'd set up the Toad a torch was shining directly at it. I crouched, frozen like a rabbit in headlights, for what felt like a full minute, heart racing. The light began pulsing in time with the thud of fast-approaching footsteps. I remembered those survival tips – 'Charge at a bull before it charges at you' and 'Make yourself bigger than an attacking bear' – and used not dissimilar logic by clambering loudly out of my tent and making my presence known. As I stood to face the light I stretched my hand out in front of my eyes and made out three silhouetted figures approaching me.

Please, please don't beat me up and steal my things.

When the figures got a little closer, however, I noticed little squares on their clothing that were reflecting the moonlight.

'Good evening, sir.'

The police. My anxiety switched gears, along with my tone.

'Good evening,' I said obediently.

Please, please don't tell me to pack up my things and move.

'Is this your tent?'

'It is. I didn't see a sign that said I couldn't pitch it here,' I said, with some truthfulness.

The three of them looked at each other. 'We were just

138

discussing that. We're not actually sure if it's permitted or not,' one of them said, to my surprise.

I couldn't see them, as the torchlight was shining unhelpfully in my eyes, but I decided that the thing to do would be to launch into my 'story'. If they weren't too old school in their attitude towards drifters, there was a chance they might let me stay. After the usual 'Wow!' and 'Amazing!' responses, the most talkative of the three announced that I was OK to camp there and that they would even 'Keep an eye on things for me.'

After they'd left I dived back into my tent, grabbed my wallet and phone, zipped it up and bounced back up the steps with full confidence in Pembroke's finest, through the crowds and towards the toffee-apple stand. Afterwards, I wandered around the fair, picking the last of the toffee out of my teeth, sizing up the tin-can shooting and the hoopla. I felt so content and, wanting to revel in it a little longer, let myself be drawn into the nearest pub and spent an hour or so sitting at the bar, chatting to the old blokes and drinking several pints of the recommended local ale.

When I returned to my tent the first thing I noticed was that the police – *my guys* – weren't watchfully guarding my things. The second thing I noticed was that my tent door was open, and the third thing I noticed was that it was completely empty. My pack, which had *everything* in it, was gone. My heart dropped. I scoured the surrounding bushes desperately, hoping for I'm not sure what, and then I began to panic. My sleeping bag, my clothes, my maps, my spare phone – my *everything* was in that pack.

I tried to think straight, about which way I would start walking to look for my stuff, but all I could think about was how much time and money this was going to cost me and how unequivocally fucked I was. My panic quickly turned to anger: firstly at myself for camping in a fucking park, then at whoever had found my tent and helped themselves to my things, and finally to the town of Pembroke for seducing me with toffee apples and assembling the crappest police force in Wales to watch over the fair. I was close to boiling over and, not knowing what else to do, I dragged the pegs out from the ground, gathered my tent up into my arms and stomped back up the steps and into town. I found myself back at the pub.

'Back already?' one of the locals said cheerfully as I rustled through the door. I felt like picking up a pool cue and throwing it at him.

'Everything all right, mate?' said the bartender, who, unlike her herd of patrons, had accurately read the expression on my face.

Through exasperated breaths I told her what had happened. The old boys at the bar chimed in uninvited with unhelpful sentences like 'Yeah, you don't want to be leaving your stuff lying around here.'

'Wait there a minute,' said the bartender. About a minute later she returned.

'We have rooms upstairs,' she said. 'You can stay here tonight if you like.'

I nodded despondently. I was grateful, but taking that room confirmed the reality of what was going on. I followed her up the stairs, my tent balled up and rustling in my hands, and into a room with a number 1 on the door. Inside was a single bed, a small TV, a kettle and a few packets of single-serving biscuits. In different circumstances, I might have been excited by the modest level of comfort on offer but, after what had happened, the room looked really sad and depressing.

I dumped my tent on the floor and lay on the bed with a

sigh. In a vague attempt to do something about the situation I decided to post about what had happened on Facebook. The following day, as I kind of thought I would, I opened Facebook to a bombardment of notifications. My post, which had detailed all the events of the night before, had been shared over a thousand times during the night. It had, to my genuine surprise, reached Facebook users in South Wales, who, after sharing, had fired a few digital shots at the town of Pembroke. I scrolled down the scores of comments to see if anyone had actually found or had seen my stuff. No luck. I went downstairs and out the back entrance of the pub and headed into town, to the park, so I could have a proper look around. As I marched along the high street I noticed one or two lingering stares coming my way. I hunted around for my pack, in the drizzle, for two and a half hours before giving up. When I walked back up the high street I was stopped by a couple who asked if I was 'the walker guy who had his stuff nicked'. I was so stunned I almost said no. I couldn't believe they recognized me from something I'd posted not even twenty-four hours ago. When I got back to the pub I checked Facebook again. There were plenty more shares, and more scathing comments about the town. After scanning through them all again, I eventually read this:

'Jake, we think we know where your stuff is! Give us a call!'

At first I thought it was a wind-up. But when I checked my inbox I had an unopened message from the same user, along with their phone number. I called it. The person who answered sounded excited to speak to me and said that she'd seen what looked to be a load of camping stuff in a bush near her house. She offered to come and pick me up so I could check if it was mine.

With some hesitation but no other play, I accepted, and an

hour later I was in the car of yet another perfect stranger, off to go and look at a hedge. When we arrived I spotted what looked like my sleeping bag on top of a bed of stinging nettles. I jumped out of the car to have a closer look, and there it was, sitting as perfectly as a pearl. I looked a little further down and there was my pack, all its contents strewn around it. It seemed that someone had seen my post and decided to lob it somewhere relatively public so someone would find it. Relief engorged me. It was all there, every item, and once it was all safely back in my pack I ran over to my driver and hugged her.

Most people I spoke to about the incident in Pembroke were embarrassed that I got robbed in their town and worried that the experience would tarnish my opinion of the place. To the contrary, I think I'll remember Pembroke as the town that rallied together and got me my stuff back after one little shit stole my things. The power of a tight-knit community is a beautiful thing, and there was a very real power of community, it would seem, in South Wales.

I posted again on Facebook to tell everyone that I'd been reunited with my things, only a day after losing them. As a direct result of taking to social media, I received countless more donations for the Mental Health Foundation, and people were beginning to talk to each other via my posts about their mental health. What began as an absolute nightmare had somehow made everything better, to the point where I almost felt grateful to the person who had ransacked my tent.

Of course I was a bit more cautious after that, camping smart, but I tried also to remain trusting of the people I encountered. Human interaction, as I've said before, is so unbelievably crucial to feeling good. Feeling like you belong, like you're part of the fabric of society, helps restore a sense of worth. At least, to me it does. It's important to remember that while we're all different, we're all on the same team, especially when times get hard for those around us. Being kind and helping your fellow human is one of the best things you can do for your mental health, because it's what we're built to do. It's our instinct to support one another and to empathize with someone else's plight, and in doing so we have an opportunity to feel connected, to feel human, something that can sometimes cease to be when our own times get hard.

My remaining time in Wales was peaceful. I traversed the jagged coastline of Pembrokeshire in what felt like no time at all, before joining the coastal path and continuing north. It was the first time I'd felt like a real endurance adventurer, keeping my head down, pushing through miles and miles of blustery landscape every day and wild camping at the end of it. With time against me, I felt a strong urge to double down on mileage if I was going to reach Edale before finishing the walk for winter. The days were getting shorter and it wasn't uncommon for it to be dark when I woke in the morning or set up camp at the end of the day. The pain in my left side was worse; in fact, it was there all the time now. I'd wake up most nights in such discomfort that I had to stretch before going back to sleep. The ground I slept on was cold and I shivered myself to sleep some nights.

It probably sounds like a really uncomfortable time, but my spirits had never been higher. I was amazed by my resilience, and by my desire to push on through almost constant discomfort. I felt disciplined and focused and, despite the hardships, I felt like I could handle all of it. If anything, it made the whole adventure feel wilder. More survivalist. I also had a lot of good stuff to occupy my mind with – I'd get lost in daydreams about running the London Marathon, even letting myself get carried away with thoughts of running the remainder of the route around Britain when I returned to it, just like Simon Clark.

By the time I reached Snowdonia a couple of weeks later, though, I felt ready to take a break. Not through fatigue or being fed up or feeling uncomfortable particularly, but because I was excited by the thought of embarking on a different kind of adventure. I didn't know what to expect from this documentary filming process, and that fired me up. The opportunity to appear on national TV as a mental-health advocate, to spread a message I believed in so much on a national scale, excited me. The thought of getting a London Marathon medal excited me. And after deciding that Brighton was where I wanted to hunker down for those six months while all this was going on, the thought of being near my friends when I felt this good *really* excited me.

It's one thing missing people, but when you can't relax around your friends like I sometimes can't, the feeling of missing people doesn't always go away after spending time with them. I never feel more lonely than when I feel like I'm missing a part of myself and, at that time, when I was walking up the west coast of Wales, I felt far less isolated and far away than some of the times I've spent in large groups of friends, crucifying myself internally for not being able to pull myself together and enjoy myself.

That said, to feel good in yourself and have friends around you is the greatest feeling and, to add further excitement, some of my oldest friends from back home had been in touch to ask if they could come out and meet me once I got to Snowdonia. The idea of seeing out the first half of my walk by climbing Mount Snowdon with a few of the old Maldon boys felt almost too perfect, and the thought of meeting them way out there made me so happy. They had hired an Airbnb about half an hour's drive from the start of the Miners' Track, one of the trails to the summit of Snowdon. Giles picked me up near Penrhyndeudraeth, a few miles east of Porthmadog, and drove me there. James and Chris were already waiting. After a lot of hugging and general boy noise the four of us got settled, ate dinner and got an early night ahead of our long walk the following day.

It felt so good to be with friends on such an epic section of my journey. The Cornish coast, the Pembrokeshire coast and everything in between had made me fall madly in love with the natural splendour of the British Isles, but nothing blew me away quite like the vastness of Snowdonia. As we drove towards Britain's second-highest peak the mountains looked still, but alive, like sleeping giants, and the roads that wound through their bases only served to accentuate their enormity.

We arrived at around 10 a.m. and began our ascent. I hadn't done much of this sort of thing with my friends before; it was different, but it felt good, and far healthier than the ways we used to spend our time together. From the peak of Snowdon you can clearly see the isle of Anglesey, some thirty-five miles away. In the other direction the land looks like waves forming in the sea, miles and miles of brown swells that stretch far into the distance. It's a truly awesome sight.

As I sat there with my friends, gazing silently into the distance, I couldn't help but reflect on what was happening to me. Just six months ago I'd felt so alone I could barely get out of bed, and now here I was, standing on top of one of Britain's highest mountains with old friends. It made me realize that climbing a mountain was nothing compared to climbing out of the black hole I'd fallen into earlier that year, and that, if I could do that, I could do anything.

*

The next morning, before we parted, Giles insisted on dropping me off somewhere so he and I could catch up properly. I've known Giles since we were twelve years old and, while it amused me to watch him tormentedly trying to get his head around the 'frankly colossal' distance I had walked by that point, our 'catch-up' was one of the most sincere and heartfelt conversations he and I had ever had. You get to a point with certain friends where catching up doesn't really happen anymore and you just pick up where you left off. But once in a while an old bond can be strengthened by simply checking in and seeing how you are both doing, even if it doesn't feel entirely natural. Sometimes it just feels good to know your mates still care about you.

Giles dropped me off near Wrexham, five miles or so west of the English border. Technically, he had chopped three or four days of walking off my journey, but that didn't matter. It was nothing in the grand scheme of things, and I got far more from spending quality time with my friend than I would have by walking forty miles on my own. The walk had become less about the physical challenge and more of an exploration of myself, of friendship, of humanity and life in general. As I took the road and crossed the border back into my home country, I felt like that was the perfect mindset to carry me into the next chapter.

11

I spent the next three days walking along the main road to Shrewsbury, peeling off only to find places to sleep. From there I followed the Severn Way as far as Telford before once again rejoining the Monarch's Way. As I traversed the thirty or so miles of mucky bridleways and sparse farmland of this Midlands section of the trail I cast my mind back to the day I first joined the Monarch's Way, in the lush green of the South Downs, as I attempted to navigate my and my brother's way out of Arundel. The trail felt far more picturesque in Sussex than it did in the Midlands but, after five months on the road, maybe I'd become a little desensitized to my natural surroundings, a little harder to please. I certainly felt good from being outside a lot, but that initial romance of being immersed in the British countryside felt a little lacking as I continued east and approached the outskirts of Wolverhampton. However, my sheer desire was to soak up as much of the English countryside as possible before winter pushed me on and, no matter where I was, I could feel the crisp, cool air in the morning, the smell of damp leaves, the sound of trees dancing in the breeze – every day was as calming and wholesome as I wished it to be, and it felt good to keep up a level of appreciation, especially since I wouldn't be out there much longer.

The pain in my side was beginning to become a real concern and, with filming due to begin in a matter of weeks, I felt it only right to tell the producers of the documentary. Pete, the director, booked me in for some physiotherapy appointments in Brighton. He also asked if I could go to

Bristol so I could be physically and mentally evaluated ahead of filming, and so once I reached Wolverhampton I made my way to the station and jumped on a train.

It was a typically rainy day in Bristol the day I arrived, and it made Broadcasting House feel kind of cosy, like being in the last lesson of the day at secondary school. I was met at reception by Jordan, a member of the production team, and taken to have my – slightly underwhelming – physical assessment.

My 'mental evaluation' with the show's psychologist was far more interesting. I was ushered covertly (it seemed the people taking part in the show must under no circumstance bump into one another ahead of our first official meeting) into a neglected room that felt a bit like my Year 8 form room – musty smell, worn carpet, windows so filthy on the outside you could only make out the colour of the sky from the inside. There, the psychologist and I holed up and engaged in a surprisingly candid back and forth, not just about what might be involved in the filming process but about life in general. It was like a therapy session, but with considerably less crying than in my sessions with Irene back in London. I found myself getting very real and honest with him, about my childhood, my meltdown and all kinds of things that I was, apparently, in that moment very comfortable talking about. He was only the second professional I'd ever spoken to about myself in this way, and the first I'd spoken to when I wasn't at a point of crisis. It's ironic how much easier it is to talk about the dark times when you're not in the thick of them.

Despite needing to be vocal about depression, I still find that when it actually hits me I'll do pretty much anything I can to throw people off the repulsive stench of it. Gradually, during my time filming *Mind over Marathon*, I learned more and more how to vocalize my internal voice, and every time I did it I felt more like I was picking up from where I left off. My conversation with the psychologist at the BBC that day gently nudged me towards this, and I'll always be grateful to him for the chat we had.

The next day I caught the train back up to Wolverhampton and spent my final few days on the road walking into Staffordshire. I'd arranged a place to stay with someone called Yolanda in Stoke-on-Trent, who, like Oana in Poole, I'd met through the Couchsurfing app. It was dark and a little drizzly when I arrived in the city, but I was in high spirits and keen to enjoy this last little piece of adventure before my winter break. I arrived at Yolanda's place at around 6 p.m. and was greeted with a huge smile and a freshly boiled kettle.

She was very pretty, with thick, dark hair and deep-set eyes. She was very inquisitive about my journey so far, particularly why, after walking hundreds of miles of national trails, I'd decided to come through Stoke-on-Trent. I told her I'd needed an easyish place to get back to after my winter break and that it was only about forty miles from Stoke to Edale, the village I'd originally earmarked as my mid-end point. As I spoke, Yolanda's dark eyes sparkled; I revelled in her enthusiasm, realizing just how much I was going to miss all this.

Both Yolanda and her other half, Chris, worked in neuroscience. She was working towards a PhD and Chris, a bona fide professor, was part of a team conducting some pretty groundbreaking research (it seemed) into curing hind-leg paralysis in dogs by – and I'm paraphrasing here, of course – extracting stem cells from the dog's nose and injecting them into the area that needs repairing, in this case the hind legs. He showed me some videos and, to my amazement, the dogs, who had been paralysed from the waist down (do dogs have waists?), were learning how to walk again. The coincidence of having had to endure nearly three weeks of intense leg pain while on a challenge I'd recently rebranded as 'Black Dog Walks' wasn't lost on me.

After a few cups of tea Yolanda suggested that the three of us head down to the local pub to take part in their weekly quiz. If I haven't already made my feelings of intellectual inferiority clear from simply trying to explain what my hosts did for a living, all you need to know is that my sole contribution to the entire quiz was the answer 'Natalie Imbruglia'. It was an evening of laughter and interesting conversation with deeply kind people, and the perfect way to stick a bookmark in my journey, for now.

After saying my goodbyes I caught the train to Maldon to grab a few things I'd need to move to Brighton and catch up with my family. It was so great to see everyone and, without really realizing it, without much in the way of ceremony, the first half of the walk was over. I would reflect on those six months in southern England and Wales a lot over the coming weeks, but my immediate feelings were almost all excitement about filming the documentary and returning, for a short while, to the East Sussex coast.

After stashing my walking clothes and camping stuff in my old room on Mum's boat I repacked my rucksack with 'civilian' items and spent a few days catching up with Mum, sharing stories from the road and taking long, wintry walks along the river with Reggie. As ever, a fleeting visit to my home town helped reset me and make me feel ready to embark on the next part of my life, and when the sea air hit me as I stepped out of Brighton station I felt ready to begin a new type of adventure.

I moved to Brighton to have a base while filming and, as fate would have it, the house I'd lived in some four years or so previously had a spare room going. I was offered a job at my friend Simon's pub, the Bottom's Rest, and with my adult responsibilities sorted within a day of arriving, I was free to relax and spend a few days catching up with friends.

Everyone seemed eager to hear about my walk, but even more keen to talk about mental health. Friends who had always seemed so confident, so together and healthy, were messaging me to see if I wanted to get coffee (a sure sign there's something fairly pressing to discuss). It felt good to be reconnected, but it also concerned me just how common it seemed to be for people to feel overwhelmed and confused by life. One thing I did notice during these meet-ups was that although everyone's stress stemmed from different sources I found myself giving out the same sort of advice – you're overloaded, take a step back, do more for yourself, knock boozing on the head . . . I recalled my brief conversation with Nancy, the traveller in Coverack, when I'd realized that, while the root cause of people's distress can vary quite drastically, the emotional response is often really similar, and perhaps the reason why so many people struggle to talk about their problems is that they focus on the external factors that caused them rather than their body's response to it. The reality is that not everyone is going to be able to relate to the things going on around you with work, at home, with your partner, etc., so it's hard to bring that sort of thing up in a way that people can understand or connect to. Your emotional response to these things, however – I feel lost, I feel angry, I feel a weight on my shoulders, and so on – people know what these things feel like and, when common ground is discovered, connections are made and problems can be properly discussed. At the end of the day, our brains are pattern-seeking machines, so when someone 'gets' what you're going through, it provides some comfort; comfort that you're not the only one struggling, that you're not a freak, that someone understands. Learning to be open in this way builds bridges, it allows you the freedom to be open, to depend on people and be OK to have them depend on you too. It provides a safe space for you to expel your darkest, least coherent, least logical narrative without fear of judgement. Over the six months I moved back to Brighton I'd learn all about the power of community, among other things, after meeting nine new people who would become friends forever.

The time came to start work on *Mind over Marathon*. We were going to be filming at Bisham Abbey, a sports complex near Windsor where some of Team GB train. I arrived on a perfect autumn morning and the early-morning sun had already begun pouring through the cracks in the trees, spilling on to the icy grass and creating ghosts that danced around the historic abbey. Four smiling members of the production team were there to greet me: Pete, Jordan, Emily and Claire.

Inside the abbey were the rest of the production team and the show's presenter, TV's Nick Knowles, who would meet and greet me and the rest of the 'unlikely runners' (as we had been dubbed) one by one. I was nervous and, looking at them, so were the other participants. None of us knew what was happening, and everyone looked either overwhelmed or incredibly uncomfortable. I remember wondering if I'd made a mistake by agreeing to take part in a documentary about mental health. Seeing how ill at ease these people were, in that moment the whole thing felt slightly exploitative, like we were being wheeled out to have our problems (in some cases, very serious problems) made palatable to the general public, and that they'd mock us as freely and mercilessly as if we were *Love Island* contestants.

One of the participants, Steve, a gentle white-haired York-shireman in his late forties, looked like he was going to throw up. When I shook his hand I felt the sweat on him and noticed that his leg was shaking uncontrollably. I felt so sorry for him, and again wondered if I'd made a seriously bad call by agreeing to be involved. I would later find out from Pete, the show's director, that the production team had agonized for weeks over how to introduce us all to each other in a way that was both respectful to our mental health and would work, compositionally, for TV. In the end they'd agreed that Nick would welcome us all in individually, and after every-one was in and introduced the filming would stop and there would be support available to anyone who felt they needed it. However, despite the palpable anxiety in the room, and how stressful that half an hour or so appeared to be for some of the participants, it all worked out OK. There were hugs and warm smiles and reassuring words and, before long, every-one seemed relaxed and, crucially, respectful. It would be the only time during the entire process I would question the intentions of the project.

As well as Steve, there was Georgie, a police officer from Tenby, in South Wales; Rhian, who had set up a charity to help suddenly bereaved families after the sudden death of her infant son and, heartbreakingly, subsequent suicide of her husband; Paul, a brewer from Yorkshire; Shereece, a pro-fessional singer and single parent; Sam, an A&R scout; Mel, a hairdresser; Claudia, a PR agent and fellow Brightonian; and Poppy, who would become a very close friend and, although she'd probably disagree with this, the glue that held the group together during filming. She'd had a difficult life and, although she was only in her mid-twenties, her eyes would occasionally let you in to the trauma she'd experienced. She was living with post-traumatic stress after her home was invaded, just like Jamie, the guy I'd stayed with in Swansea, and although very tough on the outside she could become very vulnerable and introverted at any moment. I was drawn to her from the minute I met her. Together, we made up a merry group of misfits who over the next six months would bond in a way that felt uniquely supportive and profoundly honest. The show's objective was to capture this but to also have all ten of us on the start line of the London Marathon the following April.

Running a marathon, as I would come to realize, is no joke, and the BBC had brought in the services of two coaches: Charlie Dark, who founded the London running collective Run Dem Crew, and Chevy Rough, captain of the 'mindful movement' crew Chasing Lights. Chevy would become our main coach, putting together our training schedules and introducing us to breathing and visualization techniques, while Charlie was there to offer guidance, encouragement and reassurance in the passionate and lyrical way that would become so familiar to us all. To be able to run the London Marathon without applying felt lucky enough, but to have bespoke training schedules felt like a real privilege, and one I gratefully accepted.

Since my legs were strong from the walk but still not a hundred per cent, despite the physio sessions to treat what turned out to be my ITB (iliotibial band), Chevy set me a training schedule that focused more on strengthening my core, which, although useful, didn't exactly get me pumped to begin the process. The reason I love walking and running is because I like to move through landscapes and be inspired by my surroundings. Squats, lunges and planking were, in my opinion, the antithesis of that. I was willing to get stuck in, though, and to my surprise, after only a few weeks I was already noticing the benefits. With a stronger core I was able to run with better form, keep my back nice and straight, and run with my bum rather than my hips (one of several bad habits Chevy had spotted early on and attempted to iron out).

A month into training the production team signed Claudia and me up to run the Guildford 10k together. It was the first running event I'd ever entered, and Claudia's too. When the horn sounded the start of the race I ran into the pack with confidence, like I was trying to get to the front row of a gig. In the melee I slipped on the mud, cracking my left knee hard into the ground. It hurt, but I was so embarrassed I got straight back up and continued running. I'd fallen over before I'd even run two hundred yards, thankfully without the cameras there, and put a hole in my nice new joggers.

I'd been so determined to make the rest of the race count I didn't think to check if there was any damage until I reached the finish line. Then, I pulled the leg of my joggers up. My knee must have hit a stone or a root or something when I fell, and it hadn't just cut the skin but split it. Because I'd run on it for a good hour afterwards the cut had torn open, leaving me with a very nasty-looking wound. Not that I cared. I'd just got a medal for running 10k, and something about that had flicked a switch and lit a part of me up.

Although I'd never considered myself a proper 'runner', running's always been what I've done whenever I felt like I needed some exercise. It's the closest thing to an 'antidote' for my depression. When I start to feel like a slave to my thoughts and emotions, running helps me feel free. When I have a problem, running helps me solve it. It's almost meditative, in the sense that my thoughts pass in and out very fluidly, allowing me to think clearly. Being static for a long time often makes me feel smothered and unable to escape the weight of negative thoughts; my mind feels congested. Running can sort that out too. It also just makes me happy, for a reason I still can't explain. When I see a footballer run towards the home fans after scoring a goal, I sometimes think, 'That's how I feel when I'm running.' It's the only time in my life I ever feel kind of bulletproof, like nothing can touch me. Yes, the endorphins probably have something to do with it, but for me there's something more powerful going on. It's like magic. It lifts me and allows me to communicate with myself like nothing else can. I never, ever seem to regret going for a run, even if it ends in a two-hour wait in A&E with fat dripping out of my leg. When I got over that finish line at Guildford and someone put a medal around my neck, something happened. A sense of achievement via a solid hit of dopamine, sure, but also a kind of enlightening, like everything about that moment made total sense to me.

Sitting in A&E at Sussex County Hospital, waiting for a doctor to stitch my knee, Pete asked me, 'This hasn't put you off, has it?'

I looked at my medal and replied, genuinely, 'I don't think anything could put me off running now.'

Three weeks and six stitches later my knee had more or less healed and I found myself at the start line of the Brighton half-marathon. Claudia and I had been paired up again, only this time, rather than feeling like co-participants, we now ran together as friends.

It was a damp and grey morning, but the air was full of optimism. Hordes of eager Brightonians lined the streets, waiting to cheer the 12,000 runners who'd signed up to take part. Along with Pete and the rest of the production team, Chevy had also come down to the south coast to give Claudia and me a last-minute pep talk and to cheer us on through the race. To my mild embarrassment, I had accidentally put on the form a predicted finish time of one hour thirty, which meant I was starting near the front of the pack with a lot of very serious, very skinny people checking their very expensive-looking watches every two seconds. Chev's tip for me in light of this slight fuck-up was to 'start slow and let all the athletes and people trying to keep up with the athletes run past me, and feel smarter than them for taking my time'. His advice proved invaluable when, at the five-mile point, and 'running smart' (as Chevy put it), I began to overtake a few people who had clearly underestimated the race and bolted a little too eagerly out of the blocks. It was a lesson learned the hard way for them, and I guess more vicariously for me; I actually felt a bit sick passing them, knowing they were already out of puff with eight miles still left to run. 'Slow and steady,' I remember saying to myself. 'Slow and steady finishes the race.'

I maintained my speed, as Chevy had instructed, keeping my cadence consistent and focusing on my breathing. As I crossed the twelve-mile marker I began to feel like I had a strong finish in me and, as the crowds got thicker and louder as I approached the finish, I decided to go for it. I picked my pace up as I passed Palace Pier, and when the finish line came into view I switched up one final gear. My feet pounded the concrete like a jackhammer. My eyes widened and my lungs gasped huge volumes of air in and out with every stride. Ahead of me I saw people crossing the line, and when I felt like I couldn't sprint anymore I ran even faster. The last few strides were intense, like my body was about to give out, but I made it to the line before I slowed down and finished the race in a time of 1 hour 58 minutes. I couldn't believe I'd run a half-marathon that quickly, and I fell into Pete's arms in a heap of relief and pride in equal measure.

After getting my medal I waited at the finish line for Claudia. After about half an hour I spotted her, and I couldn't contain my excitement. I couldn't wait for her to feel what I'd felt when I crossed that line, and the second she did the two of us fell into an emotional and euphoric embrace. It was one of the best feelings I've ever had. I couldn't remember ever being so happy for anyone, and in that moment I understood the magic. I wanted to carry on running forever. I felt I had achieved the mindset I needed to run a full marathon.

Our shooting schedule ramped up in the weeks leading up to the London Marathon, and so did our training. I was told I had to be doing three 5–10-mile runs a week, and one long run (which I took to mean anything over ten miles). Before each run I would go through the light stretches Chevy had taught me, along with twenty squats and twenty lunges. I would plank for three minutes in the morning and in the evening, and I used the foam roller (a horribly painful but very effective tool to aid muscle recovery) we were given on the first day of shooting before going to bed. The pain in my ITB was finally gone and I felt that was down to being diligent with the stretching schedule and finally learning how to 'run smart'.

By this time, the whole crew had become incredibly close, talking and checking in with each other regularly as friends, so regular meets were always fun and relaxed. Saying that, an important and significant day in the schedule was approaching, one that Pete had managed to keep successfully under wraps (despite a few rumours) until the night before. All we knew was that we were due to meet at St Mary's University in Twickenham to do, among other things, some running around the athletics track. I had work until 9 p.m. at the Bottom's Rest the night before and had to head straight to

Brighton station afterwards to catch the train to London. I'd suffered a minor ankle injury during my training, but I was happy to go along anyway, just to hang out with everyone, so I didn't pack any running clothes. On the way to the station I got a call from Pete.

'All set for tomorrow?' he asked.

'Yep, all set. Can you tell me what the big surprise is yet?'

'Yes. We were going to keep it to ourselves but we've realized that a few of you might feel more comfortable with some warning so, here it is . . . you're meeting the royals.'

I paused. Then: 'The royals? Which royals?'

'William, Kate and Harry,' said Pete.

I looked down at what I had on. My clothes were fresh on that day so I hadn't felt the need to pack much. In my bag was a clean T-shirt and fresh socks and underwear, but I wouldn't be able to change my jeans, which were old and had holes in, or my DMs, which were also old and had holes in. I've never been one to dress smart unless I absolutely have to – I've even slacked off at weddings before – but in that moment I felt like I just could not meet the royal family wearing what I was wearing. It must be something deeply ingrained in me, as an Englishman: one must be well presented when one meets royalty.

'I'm not appropriately dressed,' I said.

'Don't worry, we'll sort something out,' said Pete. (As was his catchphrase.)

I had to trust him and, even if I didn't, it was too late to nip home now.

The next morning I came down to breakfast at the hotel we'd all been staying at. Everyone was buzzing to meet the royals, speculating on who 'the nice one is', how they were going to greet us, and so on. My excitement, however, was slightly limited, due to the fact I was still dressed for slinging pints. Throughout the process of filming Pete had reiterated that if there was anything we ever needed, the budget would cover it. I hadn't needed or asked for anything so far, but that morning, at the risk of being seen as a diva, I was in need.

'Pete,' I said, 'I'm so sorry to ask this, but is someone able to do a Sports Direct run? I *can't* wear these jeans and these shoes to meet the royal family. My gran would kill me.'

'What size feet are you, Jake?' said a deep, booming voice from behind me.

I turned round. 'Ten and a half,' I said, to TV's Nick Knowles.

'I brought my running stuff with me, just in case. Do you want to borrow it?'

Five minutes later I was in a toilet changing into Nick Knowles's clothes to meet Prince William, Prince Harry and Kate Middleton, Duchess of Cambridge. Needless to say, the situation was more like some surreal, arbitrary dream than real life. Despite Nick's feet being, would you believe, slightly smaller than mine, his trainers just about fit. His jogging bottoms were slightly shiny, a bit like an eighties shell suit, and I loved them. The next thing I knew, we were all piling into a minibus and heading to the university and, within the hour, assembled on the 400-metre track at St Mary's, we were being introduced to some of the most recognizable people in the world.

The initial shock factor of meeting the royals is quite something. They have an air about them that's so warm and familiar, like being reunited with old family, but it's mixed with the fact that they're so famous you never really consider them to be real people. As I was being mic-ed up opposite Prince Harry, wearing TV's Nick Knowles's trainers, with an *entire* production crew filming every second of our exchange, I briefly wondered if I was living what my future self would refer to as 'the most surreal moment of my entire life'.

The Duke and Duchess of Cambridge are the patrons of

the charity Heads Together, which encourages openness about mental well-being. It was the official sponsor of the London Marathon that year, and our documentary, *Mind over Marathon*, was going to be one of the main vehicles to help drive home the message. Say what you want about the royals, but I think using their influence for a cause as universal as mental health is maybe the best show of intent ever made by a British monarchy. The more I spoke with them, the more I felt like I was really getting to know them. They were leading by example, and I was happy to follow.

We would see them again on 23 April, the day of the London Marathon.

The evening before, on the orders of my coach, Charlie, I laid my full kit out on the desk of my hotel room in Greenwich. This, I now recognize, is a bit of a pre-match ritual for some runners. You lay down everything you take with you on race day (your clothes, your shoes, your race number, etc.), take a picture and post it on social media. It's a good way to get a bunch of good-luck messages, and also to make sure you haven't forgotten anything. After I posted my 'kit lay' on Instagram my phone rang. It was Simon Clark, the man running the coast of Britain who I'd first bumped into in South Wales. Since our chance meeting in Carmarthen, Simon and I had somehow become friends – I even put him up for the night when his lap of Britain took him through Brighton and, of all the people I would have wanted to speak to ahead of running a marathon, I was touched that it was him who called. He gave me some great advice, mostly involving post-race massages, and told me some inspiring stories from marathons he had run in his younger years. When I got off the phone all I wanted was to make him proud and, in order to do that, he'd said, all I had to do was have fun.

The next morning we were taken to various sections of the site to do interviews. The first episode of *Mind over Marathon* had aired on BBC1 two nights previously and as a result we were being recognized by pretty much everybody. It was the only time in my life I experienced what it was like to feel that I was really *known*, and while, admittedly, it was a bit creepy at times, the recognition we were getting for being open about our mental health was, for the most part, very moving.

Before the race began we were once again visited by the royals. Shaking hands with HRH Prince William, a wave of nervous adrenaline hit me when I realized I'd not had a chance to wipe the vaseline off my hand, the hand I'd greeted him with and which, a minute previously, I'd used to, as I said to the Prince, 'grease up my groin'. He looked at his hand, then at me, and to my pathetic relief, he laughed.

London was transformed – people dawdling, heads raised, eye contact, smiles on faces, pockets of excited chatter. People had chosen to be exactly where they were in these moments, supporting one another; they were all present, and the resulting light and positivity was crackling in the air, infectious and inescapable.

The race itself was pure magic. Poppy and I ran, walked and chatted to people the whole way, drinking in the experience and making the most of the day, just like Simon had suggested. Most of the time I feel like life is washing over me, briefly, making no lasting impression. I sometimes feel like I have a short circuit that makes me unable to process emotion in normal time, but as I crossed the finish line of the London Marathon I was thankful that I *was* in the moment, alive with beautiful emotion. Pure, raw and true. It felt good to finally feel that.

I've tried to revisit that day and sum it up a few times since beginning to write this book, but the piece I wrote the day after the marathon still feels the most real . . .

> *As I approach the marker at mile 26 my body begins to feel heavy. It feels like with every step that I take another layer of clothing goes on. By the time me and Poppy march purposefully past Big Ben and the Houses of Parliament I feel like I'm wearing a suit of armour. And then we run. The last 0.2 miles is harder than the rest of the 26 before it put together. It's almost impossible, I feel like I keep slipping in and out of consciousness. Eight hundred metres to go . . . 600 metres . . . 400. I feel like I'm running through water. Two hundred . . . the crowd cheers as I snap back into reality and realize what's happening; where I am and what I'm about to do. I reach out and grab Poppy's hand and do my best to hold it up, but I'm so weak I can barely lift my own arm. Our feet pound the road in unison, with both our right knees strapped up, as we, 14222 and 14225, finally, FINALLY, cross the line in 5:52. And as my pace drops and I begin to walk I feel strangely calm. I glide over to the people who have been there with me over the past six months. And as I watch them cry and hug and congratulate, I take a step back and I make a promise to myself. That whenever I feel worthless, whenever I feel alone, whenever I sense that ominous storm heading my way, I will play this moment over and over in my head until it goes away. Because with the feeling I have right now, I don't want to die. I want to live forever.*

12

Being part of *Mind over Marathon*, being involved in the crea-
tion of something that reached, touched and supported so
many people, was and always will be the most extraordinary
experience of my life, so I decided to let the dust settle for a
few weeks after running the marathon before setting back
off on the walk. I was getting recognized in the street, and as
fun and humbling and dreamlike as that was for a while, I
really didn't want it to filter into the second half of my journey. I hadn't thought about it before setting off, but I'd really
enjoyed the anonymity of those first six months. Feeling like
a ghost, wandering silently through towns and villages without disturbing the lives of others, observing constantly and
interacting rarely, had had a profoundly calming effect
on me, and after being thrown back into a busy existence of
work and housemates and talking endlessly about my emotions on camera for six months I was keen to reclaim that
anonymity and calm.

Thankfully, I didn't have to wait long to stop feeling like
public property. After a fortnight of new programmes and
news items the world moved on. My fifteen minutes of fame
evaporated and I returned to life as just another guy in a cap.
It's quite a transition. That little bit of fame is like being
hooked up to a drip of pure dopamine: it gives you an intense,
sustained feeling of accomplishment. And that makes it easy
to get carried away with the whole thing, to feel like you were
right all along and that you *are* in fact the centre of the universe and that you *had* been put on earth for an important

reason. That's why I felt I had to reground myself, because that wasn't the right mindset to be heading back out on the road with.

Things had changed massively for me online. I'd gained thousands of new followers across my social media platforms, people who had seen the programme and were now contacting me for advice. It forced me to think about how to communicate with people I'd never met before about highly emotive and personal things. With no real knowledge of how to talk to people in this way and zero education to back any advice up, I struggled a little, not knowing what to do for the best. But the good thing was that it was making a previously difficult conversation that little bit more normal and relaxed. Discussing my feelings with strangers, I realized, was helping to normalize the type of language I needed to feel comfortable using when my mental health, inevitably, took a turn for the worse.

It's also really interesting to hear how other people choose to articulate their emotions; it helps to understand what it is that so many of us are going through. I decided to invite some people to do something of a 'mini-walk' with me, so I could continue learning to talk to people about mental health in new ways. I invited my friend Sam, one of the other runners in *Mind over Marathon* – 'the fit one', as many of my female friends referred to him – to meet me in Stoke so the two of us could walk towards Edale, where my walk would officially start up again.

We met up in the city centre, which I realized upon arrival wasn't quite the lush, pastoral setting Sam had probably envisaged we'd be walking through, but it was symbolic to me – Stoke was the city where the first half of my walk had ended, and it felt good to be back there with a friend. I assured Sam that it would only take an hour or two to get to 'the good stuff', and after a few uninspiring miles through the centre we found ourselves with the fields and trees of Longsdon all around us as we headed east towards Leek. Because we had lived the same 'fifteen minutes of fame' experience, there was no shortage of conversation topics. It had been an enormous experience for both of us, and now that it was all over we were able to discuss it properly and decompress. Half an hour or so before we got to Leek, however, Sam became distant. When we stopped for some water he took out his phone, and after a few minutes he asked if I'd mind if he took a bus to Macclesfield so he could grab a few supplies. Recognizing this as a sign he needed some time alone, I suggested that I continued on to Leek and find somewhere for us to have dinner, as it would probably be easier for him to get to. He agreed, and we parted ways.

I arrived in Leek shortly afterwards and found a decent-looking place to drop my bag and have a drink. At the bar I began talking to one of the staff, Amy. It wasn't long before we were discussing my walk and, after I'd told her my reasons for embarking on my challenge, her eyes widened and the conversation ramped up. She appeared as ready to talk about her mental health as I was about mine, and within a few minutes we two strangers were locked into as deep a conversation as I can ever remember having.

Amy revealed that she struggled with anorexia, which was something I knew very little about. We talked and talked, and the more I listened, the more I began to understand. She made me realize that anorexia isn't really about losing weight or achieving the perfect body, it's about regaining control, and the impulse to embark on destructive behaviours when your head is a mess was something I could definitely relate to. I suddenly wished Sam was there to contribute, and after an hour or so I rang him to see where he was. When he answered he sounded mightily pissed off.

'I'm pretty sure I've missed the last bus back to Leek.'

'Shit,' I replied, unhelpfully.

I put him on speaker and opened my map. There was one major A road connecting Leek to Macclesfield.

I told Amy that Sam was stranded and, without even stopping to think, she said, 'I'll pick him up.'

Back in Leek, the three of us spent a couple of hours deep in enlightening and moving conversation. It felt like Amy especially had a lot she wanted to get off her chest, and by the time Sam and I left it almost felt like she'd had a breakthrough. Perhaps it was a topic she'd never gone into in that much depth, or in that relaxed an environment, or maybe it was just for the ever-consistent reason that Sam and I were strangers she'd likely never see again.

However, this turned out to be the case for a much darker reason. Two weeks later I was contacted by one of Amy's colleagues, asking if I could send her the group photo I took of everyone at the pub. It turned out that it was the last picture taken of Amy alive. The very day after I'd met her, she died in a car crash.

The news hit me surprisingly hard. I hadn't even known she existed until that day I met her, but I felt like I got to know her on a more profound level than some of my actual friends, and I'd said goodbye to her that night with a sense of real hope for her, like she was ready to forgive herself for a lot of the things she'd done to herself and move on. She'd seemed content. I guess in some ways it's probably favourable to pass away when your mind is clear, but I couldn't help but feel like Amy was ready to start over but would never get the chance.

The following day Sam and I walked to Buxton via the famous Roaches ridge. From the top you can see for miles, and when we stopped there to eat I asked Sam what he thought about the concept of walking for mental health. He said that whenever he was free from distraction, the thoughts he felt he needed to address came to the forefront of his mind, and being outside was giving him the mental space he needed to process those thoughts. I agreed with him. When it was just me and the landscape I was able to do some real work on myself and as a result felt able to accept or understand my darker or more confusing thoughts a little better. The benefit from walking with someone else, however, was that we were able to voice our self-discoveries as and when they arose, and through that an opportunity to connect emerged. We discussed all of our thoughts that day, all the things we would be too distracted to think about back home – our future, our past, our parents, everything – and when our day of walking ended it felt like the two of us had grown, maybe not a lot, but enough to realize that we were far more capable of managing our demons than we'd perhaps previously given ourselves credit for.

Sam got the train home from Buxton the following day and a few new friends joined me for the ten-mile walk to Edale. Author Bryony Gordon, who I'd met on marathon day and then again at a charity event a few months previously, came up from London with her friend, model and mental-health campaigner Jada Sezer, and a guy called Pete Thompson, who I'd read about on the BBC Sport website. Pete had recently completed his own challenge of running forty-four marathons in forty-four countries in forty-four consecutive days. When I found out he'd been doing it to raise money for Mind, I felt compelled to send him a congratulatory message on Twitter, and after a few heartfelt exchanges he agreed to come and join me for a day in the Peak District. Bryony and Jada were gearing up to unveil plans to run the London Marathon the following year in their underwear to promote body positivity – another area of mental health that wasn't at that stage on my radar. Throughout the day the two of them stripped down to their pants and bras to take photos of themselves in the countryside, and the sense of empowerment it gave them was impossible to ignore. They were clearly on to something.

In Edale, after a long day's walk, the four of us treated ourselves to a pub dinner. Those three days of walking with other people were the perfect transition from doing *Mind over Marathon* back into nomadic life, the perfect reintroduction to the walk in miniature. Now it was time to go back to Brighton and prepare myself for my second leg around Britain.

Armed with some fresh perspectives and improved fitness, I repacked my rucksack and left Brighton in June 2017, exactly one year after my walk from the Palace Pier first began. After a long train journey back to Edale, I found myself once again on my own in the middle of nowhere, plotting a route on my map. As unceremoniously as my walk began, and with a feeling like it was simply 'the next day', I let go of the previous six months, reset my focus on the road ahead and, just like that, I started walking the Pennine Way.

13

All my appreciation for nature and my desire to exist out in the open had returned on my first day back, and over the following days I immersed myself in the pastoral surroundings of the Pennine Way. I peeled away from the beaten track occasionally to explore the woods, washed my feet in streams and stood still to feel the force of nature all around me. I know it sounds cheesy, but there really is no easier way to explain it – nature was once again becoming my therapy, and as the days and miles passed so did all the residual stress of city life I had accumulated over the previous six months.

I continued north through West Yorkshire. I fell in love daily, not just with the Peak District National Park but with the towns and villages I passed through. Glossop and Marsden were so quaint and grey, but in a kind of *League of Gentlemen* way, and both made their way on to the ever-growing list of places I could see myself living in some day. The people in West Yorkshire were also beginning to steal my heart a little. Listening to two old ladies waffle about everything and nothing became one of my favourite pastimes during my coffee-shop phone-charging stops. 'So I said to Lucy – you know Lucy, she was at Ron and Elaine's anniversary buffet at The Chequers and she wore that beautiful blue dress with yellow stitching; she's a vegetarian and Terry, bless him, gave her some of his quiche when he found out because he'd had too much anyway, and he's had to watch his cholesterol since he had that scare last year – well, anyway, I said to her, I said it's got to be the exact change or the machine won't start . . .' It was like a John Cooper Clark poem, but without the irony.

By the time I reached Hebden Bridge I was back in full adventure mode – grubby, sweaty and elated by small discoveries after scrambling and bouncing through the vast, craggy landscape. I stumbled across a small cabin called 'the honesty box' that had been set up, presumably, as a welcome little oasis for walkers to recharge after a long yomp in the surrounding hills. Among the treats and produce inside were trays of cakes and flapjacks, fresh eggs, a freezer full of ice cream and, of course, a lovingly stocked selection of teas and coffees. There was no one there; it was left to you to leave money for whatever you took. It was one of the most sweet and neighbourly things I'd stumbled across, and said so much about this part of England. I helped myself to a mug of soup and a quick phone charge, left a couple of quid and walked on.

I was averaging around fourteen miles a day at this point, pushing through thousands of feet of elevation change and feeling more in tune with my body than I could ever remember. I'd begun implementing all the stretching and warming-up tips I'd amassed in my marathon training, and if there was ever a moment where I felt like a section of my body was working overtime I'd take time to stop or slow down or stretch it out. My lax attitude towards the amount of stress I was putting my body under during the first half of my walk had led to an injury that had taken a month or so to heal properly. I wasn't going to make that same mistake again.

I couldn't remember ever feeling so driven or so respectful towards myself. The amount I was moving was making as profound a difference to my mental health as it was to my physical health. I cared about me. I cared what happened to me. My confidence and self-belief were riding high, my thoughts were clear and my appetite for life and experience was unwavering. I'd wake up every morning in my tent and be excited about the day, the situations I would fall into and the people I might meet.

After only a week of picking the walk back up, however, and feeling like I was right where I wanted to be, I received an unexpected email. It was from someone at Heads Together, asking if I'd be interested in representing the charity in an endurance event called Race to the Stones the following week. My reaction was also unexpected. It was so good to be back on the road that, on the one hand, I felt there was no need to do anything but carry on, but on the other, this offer seemed to fit into the overall nature of the journey. A bit like the marathon, I felt it was an opportunity to test myself, to see what I was capable of. After some deliberation I replied, agreeing to take part. Little did I know that I'd signed up to the most physically and mentally shattering three days of my life.

Race to the Stones is either a one- or two-day (depending on which way you choose to do it) 100km ultra-marathon across the ancient Wessex Ridgeway. I didn't even know ultra-marathons existed until I got the email, and while I found it amazing that this was a thing, for some reason the mileage didn't intimidate me. I'd become a confident runner during the six months of *Mind over Marathon*, and the feeling I got when I crossed the finish line in London had made me hungry to achieve more, to progress to the next level. I saw Race to the Stones as my chance to do that. London was tough, but I was amazed at how I was able to focus my mind to push through a pain barrier – I didn't think I could do that. I was beginning to see why people become running addicts – it's not necessarily the act of running that makes you feel good (although it definitely does), it's the opportunity to marvel at your biology, to push yourself beyond what you think is all you have. The daydreams of running sections of my route around the UK were coming back, but with a big rucksack in tow, I'd conceded it wouldn't be possible. Maybe that's why, when I got an opportunity to run, I took it. I would have taken it if it were two hundred miles. I was just that desperate to run.

The RTTS course begins in Lewknor, Oxfordshire, and ends at the site of one of Britain's prehistoric marvels, the Avebury stone circle in Wiltshire. Built in the Neolithic period, the stone circle is the oldest recorded megalith in the world and thought to be a site of profound religious significance by modern-day Pagans. The Ridgeway is Britain's oldest road, and passes through some of the most quintessential English countryside and open downlands in southern England; rolling green hills dominate the landscape, peppered with English oak trees, rural fields and dusty bridleways – the perfect setting for a long run.

The plan was to meet up with Team Heads Together at the start of the race, at Field Farm on the outskirts of Lewknor, on the morning of the event. While some choose to run the whole of the route, due to the setting and the distance, most people who enter walk or run the Ridgeway over two days. The plan was for Team Heads Together to do the course in two days: fifty kilometres the first day, ending up at 'base camp', where runners and walkers can eat, regroup and get some well-needed kip before setting off on a second consecutive fifty-kilometre day. The rest of the team wanted to walk both days, but I had my heart set on running.

It certainly wasn't necessary for me to compete in an event like this, when you consider the hefty mileage I still had ahead of me on my own walk, but I seemed to have a real compulsion to say yes to everything that stemmed from my decision to walk around Britain, and after running the London Marathon my thirst for new silverware (which I suppose represented the euphoric sense of achievement I'd developed a taste for) had reached critical mass.

I decided, instead of catching a train, to hitchhike to the race and rely on the kindness of strangers to get me to the start line. In case of unforeseen complications, I decided to give myself a whole twenty-four hours to make it there. I camped in a cow field just off the canal path near Gargave the night before I was due to set off, a couple of hundred yards away from the main road. I was bursting with confidence and I couldn't wait to get up the next morning and start the journey south. I set my alarm for 6 a.m.

Contrary to common belief, you can still hitchhike in Britain. I'd been doing it for a few years before this trip, to get to and from Brighton, and while I wouldn't describe myself as a veteran, I do know that there are a few things to consider when writing a sign for hitchhiking. Firstly, it should only be two or three words long – drivers have to be able to see all the information in one glance. The key piece of info is obviously your destination, or better still the direction (being less specific gives you a bit more scope). Secondly, you want to establish a playful, slightly (but not overly) colloquial and non-threatening tone that will help convince drivers who are in two minds that they'll be safe with you. This can be tricky to achieve in just one word, so it helps to add a small flourish or a symbol in one of the letters – a flower or a smiley face, for example.

That morning I decided it best to cast a wide net and kept my sign nice and simple:

'Lift? South.' And I popped a heart where the dot of the 'i' in 'lift' would go.

Once I was on the road I started thinking about where best to position myself. This is the most crucial decision. You need to be in a place where drivers can:

a) Spot you a fair distance away.
b) See you in their rear-view mirror for a good amount of time after they've passed you (a lot of the lifts I've got over the years have been from people who drove past then doubled back).
c) Pull over easily without holding up the cars behind them.

The best spot is on a long, straight, relatively busy stretch of road close to a visible turn-off or passing point. A-roads are ideal, but only during working hours. You might assume that your chances of getting picked up improve between 7 a.m. and 9 a.m., or 5 p.m. and 7 p.m., because of the extra traffic, but I can't recall ever getting a lift from someone going to or from work. If a driver's thoughts are taken up by possibly the least enjoyable feature of their lives (their job, or their commute to their job), they aren't likely to consider taking pity on some bum with their thumb out on the side of the road. And fair enough, I suppose. I'm definitely at my least considerate of other people during business hours, *especially* people I don't know.

Ideally, you want to be catching people who are on their way to or from something that's not a part of their usual routine. My brother once hitchhiked along the coast of California with the help of two separate drivers who were on their way to funerals, which isn't as shocking a coincidence as you'd think. He also ended up partying with Casey Affleck and Joaquin Phoenix that night, which is a fantastic testimony to the vastly unpredictable nature of hitchhiking but, alas, it's a story I can't steal for this book – it's too good and he might want to write his own memoir one day. Anyway, the point is, and it might sound a little insensitive, your best targets are people who are in the midst of some sort of existential extremity. Either they're slightly freaking out about something and need something to take their mind off it, or they're unsatisfied with life but open-minded enough that they're kind of desperate for some sort of new experience. In return, if you get picked up by someone going through some sort of dark, personal shit (which *is* likely), I think you kind of owe that person an opportunity to talk it through. If there's one thing I knew for sure by now, it's that people need to talk; and if there was one thing I'd learned over the past year it was that, for some reason, people don't tend to struggle opening up as much if they're talking to someone they know they're never going to see again. A brief ride in a stranger's car is kind of the perfect environment to embrace a heartfelt discussion.

It got off to an almost perfect start. I was only waiting five or six minutes before I secured my first lift. Not my record, but definitely not far off. The car came from behind me as I faced oncoming traffic. I heard the driver sound his horn and turned to see an old black BMW perform a U-turn and pull up alongside me.

'Get in, mate,' the driver said through the open passenger-side window. He looked young, maybe twenty-one or twenty-two, a little scraggy, and kind. You can normally get all the information you need by looking into someone's eyes.

'Thanks so much,' I said, unclipping my pack.

This guy, Nathan, had the air of someone who was maybe a bit of a tearaway when they were in school but was always a good, caring guy deep down. He was in the army and told me an insane story about a time he got woken up and dragged out of his tent by a hyena while on manoeuvres in Kenya. You hear some really great stories (and opinions, for that matter) when you're hitchhiking.

Nathan took me as far as he could, and then I again

positioned myself in front of a turn-off and got my sign out. The period between the end of your first lift and the beginning of your second is easily the weirdest and most unsettling. You've just been driven somewhere you don't know by someone you don't know – you are, in every geographical sense, completely lost; and if you don't want to be lost anymore, there's only one way out of it. You have to get into another stranger's car.

I managed to keep my spirits elevated while standing by the side of the road in the middle of nowhere, cars pouring out of a service station behind me, holding a cardboard once-box with a message scrawled on it in felt tip, and after twenty minutes I was riding shotgun with Alan.

Alan was one of those ageless types – at first glance I couldn't tell whether he was in his sixties and looked great for it or in his forties and looked like he'd seen some shit. He was a big guy, both in height and build, and was the proud owner of maybe seven or eight teeth that were more or less constantly on show due to the slightly gormless grin fixed permanently on his face. He'd been fishing that morning so his car was packed full of rods and nets and other paraphernalia; I assumed he'd picked me up because he'd caught a few big'uns and was feeling like he wanted to tell me all about it. As it turned out, Alan hadn't caught anything, and it transpired that he may have picked me up for an altogether different reason.

Alan, it turned out, *had* seen some shit. He used to be addicted to heroin and, like almost all addicts, had lost most of the people in his life who ever meant anything to him. Unlike most heroin addicts, however, Alan was able to come out the other side of addiction and turn his life around. He's now a mental-health nurse, specializing specifically in helping those who've fallen down the same hole he did, and is knowledgeable and incredibly passionate about his work.

It's difficult to see an upside to going through the sort of existence Alan and so many others do, but a life in which a person falls to the bottom of a well and is able to climb back out is undeniably special. When you consider that most people who use are doing so because of some deep hurt in their lives and nobody to help them deal with it, turning to heroin must almost seem like a practical solution. Imagine that.

To the average person, a heroin addict is the lowest of the low. Trash. A scumbag. A muddy footprint on an otherwise sparkling kitchen floor. Why? Why do people see the most desperate and impoverished members of society as parasites? They're *you*, in other circumstances. They had a childhood and friends and a favourite meal and a wedding to go to and a shower that didn't work properly and maths homework and a T-shirt they loved and a first kiss and a secret that only one other person knew, and dreams and nightmares and a continual, uncontrollable series of events, situations and influences that has shaped them into the person they became, just like you. If you think heroin addiction is an indulgence, that the person you saw down an alley at 1 p.m. with a needle in their arm is just hunky dory where they are, then I'd argue that you are seriously disconnected from humanity and recommend you change this by having a five-minute conversation with someone who's lived a life like that. It doesn't matter how different you think you are to the homeless or addicts; the truth is, you aren't. They are as much a product of their past as you are, and if I somehow found myself in the position they find themselves in every day – waking up covered in my own piss, clucking for a drug that's the only thing that helps me forget my pain, a drug I'm probably forced to degrade myself daily to pay for, then that one person who treats me like a human being, who decides to have a conversation with me rather than grimace in my general direction as they pass me in the street, might make me feel like, actually, it's not all completely fucked, that I'm still part of the fabric of society and that there's a small chance I can still enjoy the only life I'll ever be given.

The world needs people like Alan. People who've been through the absolute worst and come out stronger the other side. People who take every opportunity they get to help another human being because they know how badly they've let people down in the past. People who you just know won't give up on another person when everyone else in their life has. People like Alan can inspire us. They can remind us that we're all on the same team, and that humanity may well feel like it's fucked sometimes, but it's still worth fighting for.

Alan drove me down the M6 as far as the Keele south-bound services, just outside Stoke-on-Trent, ridiculously far out of his way, of course.

Standing at the exit of a service station isn't a bad place to get picked up. The 10mph speed limit seems to give drivers that little extra time to think, and gives you the opportunity to lock eyes with them as they pass you. If you're thinking that what I'm doing there is trying to guilt the drivers into giving me a lift, you'd be absolutely right. Desperate times call for desperate measures; you just have to make sure that whoever ends up picking you up doesn't regret that decision, and then you're all square.

After ten minutes of hovering by the exit with my sign I was startled by an excitable young woman with bright electric-blue hair leaning out the passenger side of an old Mk3 Fiesta as it whizzed past me. She shouted something I couldn't make out then pointed towards the car park. And so I became acquainted with Lisa and David, a wonderfully quirky daughter–father duo heading back to their hometown after some time away together.

I loved them immediately. Lisa was 'positive energy' per-sonified and David seemed like the most laid-back person in the entire world. They were stopping for a coffee before they completed their journey and asked if I fancied joining them.

'Sure, erm . . . you're giving me a lift afterwards, though, right?' I said.

The three of us got a coffee and found a seat. At this point I felt like this had been quite a smart move by my new chums – grab a coffee with the hitchhiker first to see if he's a freak before we let him in our car. I told them about my reasons for walking around Britain and in turn Lisa was very honest about her own struggles. I was touched by how freely she could do this in front of her father. Their relationship reminded me a lot of me and my mum's; they communicated in a way that suggested they were not just parent and child but good buddies too, no topic off the table.

Sadly, Lisa and David couldn't take me very far. They dropped me at the next services and waved me off as excitedly as they'd picked me up. Lifts like that are so important for keeping your spirits elevated while you're hitchhiking, which I needed – I was beginning to get a bit conscious of time. It was nearly 6 p.m., and I'd only made it about halfway. For the first time that day, I was beginning to get a bad feeling.

I waited an hour: nothing. Another hour. Some hippy driving to Bristol came over to give me a piece of paper with a stupid Buddhist chant on it that was supposed to bring me luck. A third hour. Still nothing. It felt like my winning streak had come to an end. In the end, I waited until 11 p.m. and gave up. I wasn't going to make it.

I peered around the car park, wondering what my next move was. I spotted a grass verge that separated the car park from the main road, trudged over, climbed the verge, unclipped my pack and let it fall to the ground. All of a sudden, I had no energy. Frustrated and crestfallen, I began the process of taking everything out of my bag and setting up the Toad. I started thinking about what I should do tomorrow morning. Admit defeat, turn round and hitchhike back to Skipton? Race to the Stones started at 8 a.m., so even if I set my alarm for six and managed to get an immediate ride all the way there, there was still no guarantee I'd make it on time. Or should I plug on? Get there a little bit late, maybe catch the final wave and start the race at the back of the pack? This was probably the best-case scenario, and it was doable (technically) provided I set off very, very early.

I slumped into the Toad and thought about where I was and what was going on. I couldn't believe it: I was sleeping in a tent, illegally, at a service station. It didn't feel like 'part of the experience' anymore. This wasn't the behaviour of a normal person. This wasn't even the behaviour of a person walking around Britain to raise money for charity. This was the behaviour of a slightly organized homeless person. But I felt I couldn't turn back. That would mean it had all been for nothing.

I set my alarm for 5 a.m. Just five hours of quality service-station sleep before I'd have to get up and begin another stint of hitchhiking, and then no rest time before I began running the Wessex Ridgeway.

'It'll be over at some point,' I thought. 'I'll get there, I'll do the thing, and then it'll all be over.'

It was a defeatist pep talk, but a pep talk nonetheless. I liberated some tissue from my wash bag and stuffed it in my ears to drown out the sound of the road, lay still and closed my eyes.

BAD-ABA-DEEPBAD-ABA-DEEPBAD-ABA-DEEP!

Ugh.

I turned my alarm off and sat bolt upright. I felt like I'd only been asleep half an hour. I unzipped the tent and stared blankly at the car park before me. From all those perfect mornings waking up in fields or woods or by the sea . . . to this. What a shithole. I packed up, went into the services, bought a cup of coffee then headed back to my spot at the exit. It was just before six. Two hours until the start of the race.

A minute or two later a car sped past me, beeping its horn. I turned around and gazed with pathetic gratitude as it pulled on to the hard shoulder and put its hazards on. I ran as fast as I could, down on to the motorway and to the car. I frantically swung the rear passenger door open, peered in and saw two young lads sitting in the front.

'You legends!' I squealed.

I hurled my pack on to the back seat and dived in after it. I couldn't believe my luck. But as I continued to heap praise upon my new heroes, they remained oddly silent. 'Must be waiting for a safe moment to pull out,' I reasoned, and set about buckling myself in. As we pulled away I caught a strong, sweet smell, a smell I knew well, and not a great smell in a car. My skin went cold and prickly. Booze. And not the refreshing aroma of a freshly opened bottle of Stella but the potent sickly-sweet stench of an all-night drinking session. I leaned forward to get a better look at them.

'Are you two all right?' I said.

Silence from the one on the passenger side. 'Aghhsorryyy . . . I . . . pfffff,' the driver said.

I'd served enough pissheads in my time to see that this guy was wasted.

'OK, mate, you're gonna have to pull over and let me out,' I said.

'You what?'

'This is me. I only needed to get a bit further – you can drop me off here,' I said, a little more desperately.

He put on his indicator and pulled over and I swung the door open and jumped out, grabbing my bag and slamming the door behind me.

Hitchhiking tip: if someone pulls over, don't just get in. You aren't obliged to accept every lift you're offered. If something feels amiss, politely decline and wait for the next one.

For a second I thought about taking the number plate down and informing the police, but instead I was forced to act on my new, arguably even more dangerous reality . . . I was now standing on the hard shoulder, a blizzard of cars tearing past me. What was I going to do?

For a moment I just stood there.

Fuck.

A car sped past me, beeping its horn furiously. Then another. Then another. One driver stared at me with pure rage on his face while mouthing something sweary that I couldn't make out. I turned to look at the sign that bridged the road. It read:

'PEDESTRIAN ON MOTORWAY. REDUCE SPEED NOW.'

For what felt like the tenth time in about five minutes my guts dropped and a wave of panic engorged my body. This was bad. I couldn't remember the last time I had experienced fear like it. It was an all-over-body fear that had attacked my nervous system. I was shaking.

Vehicles continued to tear past me, drivers honking and yelling expletives. I instinctively climbed the small grass verge beside me towards the hedgerow that divided the road and Christ knows what beyond it. I stopped at the hedge, got my phone out and opened up my Ordnance Survey app. I established my location and zoomed in to try and make out what was on the other side. To my relief, the map showed a green area with no contour lines, which I knew indicated a flat, grassy area. I removed my pack and, using its and my weight, flattened a me-sized section of the hedge and fought my way through. Twigs cracked as leaves awoke and swarmed around me like bees. Thankfully, it wasn't a particularly thick hedge, and in less than a minute I'd hacked my way through to the other side.

The relief was short-lived. I still didn't know where I was or how I was going to proceed. I spent a few minutes studying my map. I had to get out of here, but I also had to find some roads to continue hitchhiking on. Apart from the motorway, I could only see winding B-roads. Pickings were slim, but I chose the best road from a bad bunch and headed towards it. I was angry, but more determined than ever to get to the start line and make this complete nightmare worthwhile.

I passed through a couple more fields and one or two narrow pathways, then found the road. For hours, I walked along winding country roads, sticking out my thumb every time a car approached me from behind. It was beginning to feel like being picked up was an impossibility. By the time I reached a busier road, it was 9 a.m. The race had begun, and I was still so many, many miles away from the start line.

However, one good thing was that, now I didn't have to stress about arriving on time, my focus pulled on solving my immediate problems. I pushed on, sticking to the main roads connecting the small towns and villages. At one point I passed the carcass of a half-burnt dog by the side of the road. My fondness for humanity and faith in people was now in freefall. At about two o'clock, after hours of walking, I spotted a car up ahead with its hazards on. I approached and the middle-aged couple in it pointed to the back seat. I was overcome with relief and gratitude as I once again slid my bag on to a random back seat and climbed in after it.

'My god. Thank you so much,' I said.

'No problem,' the man said.

'Where are you heading?' the woman asked.

'I need to get on to the M40, so maybe a service station along there?'

They weren't heading on to the M40 but agreed to take me as far as a junction or roundabout that would get me on to the motorway. At this point I was just happy to be moving quicker than three miles an hour, and graciously accepted.

I told my saviours Val and Pat all about the walk.

'Fascinating,' said Pat. 'An old friend of mine from school is doing something similar – I think he's *running* the coast of Great Britain, though.'

Surely not.

'His name's not Simon Clark, is it?'

'That's him! You know him?'

Yes! I'd followed him on Facebook, bumped into him in South Wales; he'd stayed with me in Brighton, called to wish me luck the day before the marathon.

Pat went on to tell me that he hadn't been surprised when he'd heard what his old schoolfriend was doing. 'He was always a bit different,' he said. 'I always knew he'd end up doing something mad like that.'

I wondered if any of my old schoolfriends would say the same about me.

Pat and Val cheered me up hugely and dropped me off at a road with a roundabout with an exit to the M40. I re-folded my cardboard sign to make more space. I was close enough now to write exactly where I needed to get to, which made me feel like the end was almost in sight: 'Lift? M40. Lewknor.'

Half an hour passed. There was a lot of through traffic but, so far, nobody had looked interested in stopping. Another half-hour. A car pulled up beside me and for a moment I got excited.

'Oi, are you Black Dog?' the driver yelled to me through the open window.

'Er, yeah, I guess.'

'Love it, mate, you're a legend. Keep going!' he yelled, and drove off before I got a chance to ask him for a lift.

I waited there for another hour and a half, and still nobody was stopping. I was beginning to take it personally. I started pacing up and down, muttering to myself and even hurling abuse at cars as they passed without the drivers giving me a glance. I didn't even care at this point how mental I looked. I was in a rage, and the thought that I might not make it to the start line even today was becoming a very real possibility.

After two hours, the rage had passed and in its place the familiar feeling of deep, dark sadness bedded down and prepared to cloud my every thought. Hello, old friend.

In my experience, the timing of depression can feel both random *and* circumstantial. Being able to determine if your depressed state is kind of your own fault is critical, but difficult. Difficult, because depression has a wretched habit of making you believe it's *always* your fault; critical, because by attaching a tangible reason to your drop in mood, you might be able to identify what you need to bring yourself out of it. Again, this isn't always easy. There are some problems that can only be corrected by something you're physically unable to get. Money problems, for example, can only be solved by acquiring money. However, feelings of tiredness or lethargy – fairly common things that often make me feel useless and depressed – are often a result of what I've been eating, lack of exercise or how much sleep I'm getting, and when I sort these things out those feelings usually subside. Looking objectively inward is something I've only learned to do recently, and I'm certainly no expert, but what I do know is when I'm able to counteract depressed emotions with a conscious adjustment, it really makes me feel more in control, and feeling like I'm in control often makes me feel better too.

Now, standing on the side of the road, I was hit by all the usual soundbites of depression – *Look at you, you idiot! Why do you consistently make such poor decisions? You're going to need someone to hold your hand your entire life* – but through all that internal bullying I was able to pick out a small, quiet voice right at the back. A calm, friendly voice that told me to stay calm, that it would all be fine, that this ordeal would all be over the second someone picked me up – and they would. I just had to be patient.

At about half past six, a car finally pulled up alongside me. The driver was a very neat and professional-looking young man. Tired and downcast, I peered through the open window and forced a smile.

'Thank you for stopping,' I said. 'Are you going on to the M40?'

'Erm, yes,' the man said. He seemed incredibly hesitant, like he might take some convincing before he let me in.

'I'm trying to get to Lewknor, but if you're not going that far it'd be really helpful if I could get to a service station along the way.'

'Right.' I could see in his eyes how conflicted he was. He clearly felt bad for me, he wanted to help, but he also knew he was taking a risk by letting a stranger into his car. I had to up my game a little.

'I've been standing here so long, mate. Look, I can see you're a little uncomfortable, and that's totally understandable. If you can just take me to the next services, I'll be fine from there. Would that be OK?'

Reluctantly, he agreed. Relief washed over me like a cool breeze on an uncomfortably hot day. Sitting in a car had never felt so good. The radio was tuned into a station that I imagined has the word 'Smooth' in it – Lighthouse Family, Simply Red, Des'ree – the type of music I'd usually scoff at, but in the warmth and safety of the passenger seat, and in the context of the man's crisp white shirt and glasses, I found it all very soothing; it was almost like a friend's dad had picked me up.

He took me about six miles and dropped me at the services. I got out, made for the exit and, for what I hoped would be the final time, held up my sign. I must have looked more approachable than before, as after only five minutes a car stopped and the driver beckoned me over.

'Where are you heading?' I asked.

'London,' he said.

'Can you take me as far as Lewknor?'

'I don't know where that is, but if it's on the way I'll drop you off wherever.'

Thank fuck. This was it. This horrendous day was about to come to an end.

I climbed in, thanking the driver, and as we got on to the motorway I closed my eyes and allowed every last ounce of stress to evaporate out of me.

He dropped me on the hard shoulder just before the turn-off to Lewknor. Not the safest place, but certainly not as dangerous as the hard shoulder on the M6. I got out, hopped over the barrier, descended a steep bank and joined the quiet back road below. I had a little walk ahead of me, maybe twenty minutes or so, but I didn't care. I plotted my route through a decidedly more pastoral setting and in what felt like no time at all I arrived, tired, but feeling a sense of accomplishment at having reached what would have been the bustling start point of Race to the Stones, at Field Farm, Lewknor.

*

At 7.30 p.m. Field Farm was like a ghost town. Empty barns loomed like castle walls and the dust on the ground, still warm from all the people there that morning, danced weightlessly around my boots. My hitchhiking odyssey had come to an end. It had been an experience . . . but I'm not sure it was the best experience to have before doing my first ever ultramarathon. But where was the start line?

I plodded through the farm, but saw only barns full of parked cars. I spotted a man in a hi-vis jacket, presumably the attendant, and went up to him. There was a vague look of relief on the man's face; it was clearly a lonely job.

I told him that I was registered, and about my journey, finishing with: '. . . basically, about thirty hours' hitchhiking. Unbelievable.'

'Fuck's sake. Doesn't anyone pick people up anymore? I'm Mike, by the way,' he said, and we started walking towards the start line.

'There's no signs, they've taken them all down. Everyone's gone,' he went on.

Things weren't looking good. The light was beginning to fade. I felt for my head torch. I was going to have to pull an all-nighter if I was going to get a break, a snack and a snooze at the halfway point. I was beginning to feel anxious, so I started talking to try and keep it at bay and, again, found myself telling the story of the walk. I'd told it so often now that I felt almost fake, regurgitating the same old soundbites to describe my mental health. Sometimes, however, often when the person I was speaking to had experienced a dark period in their life, the conversation opened up and took a different turn. Mike, I was about to discover, had been through the worst.

His son, Tom, had passed away a few years earlier. Mike had been overwhelmed by grief and was unable to cope with the loss. He became so unwell that he was eventually detained under the Mental Health Act; in his words, he 'turned into one of those vegetables that just sits and stares at the wall all day'. Mike's story moved me deeply. I found myself admiring how cheery and engaged he appeared that day, having experienced such profound loss so recently in his life. Sadly, as is far too common, things weren't quite what they seemed.

As I write this in a coffee shop in Brighton, two years on, I have tears in my eyes. A moment ago I went to send Mike a message on Facebook, to see if he'd mind being written into this book. Going on to his page, it became clear through the posts on his timeline that Mike passed away about a year after I'd met him. After a bit of digging I found the coroner's report, which confirmed my worst fear: Mike had taken his own life. I tracked down his daughter on social media and sent her my condolences, telling her that I'd never have been able to do what I did on the day I met him without his help. It makes me so sad to know that his grief was what killed him. He was a good person, a kind person, and I'm sure his family miss him deeply.

That evening, I'd intended to hide my pack in a hedge or somewhere (when will I learn?), but Mike wasn't having any of it. He insisted we exchange numbers and said he'd hang on to it and keep it safe. I retrieved the things I needed to get me to the halfway point, which is when I realized one of my water bottles was missing. It must have fallen out in someone's car. So with one full water bottle, a head torch, my phone and my sleeping bag (but no backpack, so I'd have to carry everything in my hands), I walked towards the row of trees that marked the start point.

'There are plenty of taps to fill your bottle up from on the way, just keep your eyes peeled,' Mike called out, and then, almost thirteen hours after the race had officially begun, I headed off from the start line.

It's fair to say that I'd been focusing so hard on getting here I hadn't given much thought to the race itself, and I'd savagely underestimated the distance. A hundred kilometres – that's sixty-two miles, or roughly the equivalent of two and a half marathons, and I was going to have to run the first fifty kilometres in the dark.

However, for some reason, thinking about the distance didn't affect me negatively. Maybe it was because, after two days standing by the side of the road with my thumb out, I was just excited to be there. I felt an intense surge of exhilaration bordering on delirium, and let out several loud howls as I set off.

Normally in a trail-running event like RTTS there are markers and way points that guide the runners through the course. Seeing as I'd started half a day behind the back of the pack, they'd all been taken down, so all I had were wooden signposts and my Ordnance Survey app. Acutely aware that I wouldn't be able to charge my phone over the coming thirty-six hours, I switched to flight mode and followed the GPS through the woodland that makes up the first five or six kilometres of the Ridgeway. The sun was beginning to set and, way before I thought I was going to, I started losing light. I felt a wave of panic, remembering that my head torch had turned itself off while I was setting up my tent three nights previously. I clicked the on switch just in case and, to my complete lack of surprise, nothing happened. This was a real problem. There was no way I could navigate, let alone run fifty kilometres, in total darkness. I was going to have to stop and find somewhere to sleep until the sun came up and then attempt the unthinkable – run the entire course in one day. Thankfully, after another few minutes of literal blind panic, the trail fed out into a meticulously manicured lawn. Usually, I'd shudder at the sight of a country club, but considering the predicament I was in, I was pleased to stumble across it, as it might offer something other than bare ground to sleep on. After a quick look around, I clambered into a stray golf buggy and wedged myself into my sleeping bag. A rough and fidgety night lay ahead, but I did my best to get cosy enough so I could nod off quickly. I was shattered. The last two days had caught up with me, and I'd run perhaps seven or eight k, which in the grand scheme of things was nothing. It meant I would have to attempt the remaining ninety k plus in one hit. I didn't know if that was even possible, but I was here now and I was determined to give it a go. I took my phone out, checked the map one last time and set my alarm for 4 a.m.

The dawn hadn't quite set in when my alarm went off, but there were sporadic grey patches poking through the black sky that suggested it wouldn't be too long before I had enough light to push on. I sat silently for ten minutes, allowing the emerging light to reveal the landscape. I watched my breath condense into clouds as tiny beads of condensation rolled lazily off my sleeping bag. I fought a brief early-morning urge to snuggle up and warm myself through and a few moments later I was up and out of the buggy, stuffing my sleeping bag back into its case and attempting to warm myself up by doing star jumps. The air was cool and there was a slight breeze: perfect running conditions. After a diligent ten minutes of warm-ups and stretching, I checked my map to determine which direction I should be heading. I felt like an orienteering group leader with no group, and I was about to attempt to run sixty miles in a day. It was insane, but something was driving me and I felt sure that, as long as I ignored every instinct to give up, I would get through it. My phone was down to 39 per cent battery. I clutched my water bottle and my sleeping bag, filled my lungs with a few deep breaths, and began to run.

Without meaning to sound like a dick, the first fifty k was surprisingly doable. The Ridgeway is mostly flat, and the surrounding Chilterns landscape is teeming with pastoral views of vast woodland and rolling green fields, a wonderful setting for a long (OK, *very* long) run. I think that a slight, unconscious tweak in my mindset had also occurred; knowing I had two and a half marathons to run somehow made running the first one feel almost easy. I remembered feeling something similar at the halfway point of the London Marathon, amazed at how much I still had in the tank after feeling absolutely done in after covering the exact same mileage at the Brighton half-marathon. It's like my mind had worked out for me that it's not the distance itself that determines how tired I get but the travelled mileage relative to the overall distance. I was aware of the immense physical suffering my body was going to go through that day, so it was encouraging to realize that my subconscious pit crew were busy behind the scenes doing relativity sums as a way to help ease the prospect of running such an insane number of miles.

It worked wonders for the first fifty k, until I reached base camp, only to discover that everything had been packed away, and the hearty sustenance and lashings of cold beverages I had been fantasizing about for the past six hours had been either consumed or binned. I'd already eaten the three cereal bars I had on me and had finished my litre of water an hour before I got to the halfway point. I was hungry. And thirsty. And pissed off. And worried. If I didn't eat something and get rehydrated before I ran 50k all over again, I might not make it to the end. And if I didn't make it to the end, I might not get a lift back! On any other day, this would be the moment I cut my losses and tried to hitch a lift with one of the people packing the area down, back to the start line so I could grab my pack off Mike and call it a day. But there was still something deep inside me, a voice that was telling me that if I kept going I was going to finish this race. But in order to do that I absolutely *had* to eat.

I approached one of the officials who was still there and explained the situation. Perhaps sensing that I was one inconvenience away from throwing an enormous wobbler, the man nipped off to 'see what he could do' and returned five minutes later with some crisps, some Wagon Wheels, two cold bacon sandwiches and three litres of water. I was saved, and in no time at all I had polished off the snacks, downed some of the water and used the rest to fill my bottle up. I thanked the angel man who had sorted me out and fifteen minutes after eating I rejoined the Ridgeway, only this time walking, so as not to get a stitch.

My phone was now at 21 per cent. While I still had a strong feeling I was going to make it, I was now not too confident I would get there before everyone had packed up and left. I wasn't sure if the organizers even knew I was in the race – I hadn't registered at the start so I didn't have a race number or anything, and although I'd tweeted the event organizers to tell them there was 'a runner coming up the rear', I wasn't sure if anyone had seen it. I decided I probably needed to take my phone off flight mode so I could check Twitter and message Sofia, my contact at Heads Together, who was, presumably, already a whole bunch of kilometres ahead, to ask if she could wait for me. Then I put my phone back on flight mode – battery 15 per cent – and began to run.

What happened over the course of the following ten hours – and I'm not exaggerating – was a subtle blend of physical torture and temporary insanity. After another four hours of running, sitting down, running again, my phone was dead. My pace had probably halved due to the blisters that had formed during the first 50k, which were now tearing open one by one inside my shoes. My legs felt like they had drunk every millilitre of blood from the rest of my body and, to cap it all, I was very, *very* hot.

An hour later I began dreaming while I was running. This, again, is not an exaggeration; I slipped away so deeply into random thoughts that I was beginning to see them with my eyes open. Whether these were simply incredibly vivid images in my head or I was fully hallucinating, I'm not sure, but I was catching myself communicating with people who weren't there and losing my grip on what was real and what wasn't. Part of me, the part of me that loved to take psychedelic drugs in my twenties, was enjoying the hallucinations. There were balloons and people I went to school with and animals and all sorts of fun things going on around me. The other side of me, however, the side who didn't want to die, was beginning to get concerned. I slowed right down to a walk, then stumbled and collapsed on to all fours, before finally laying flat out on the grass beside the track. I fell into a deep sleep, deep enough to have dreams that had proper beginnings, middles and ends.

I woke some time later. I have no idea how long I slept. It could have been ten minutes or two hours, but it was what I needed. After a few hazy moments I remembered where I was, what I'd got myself into, and what I had to do. There was no point in turning back at this point because there would be nobody left at base camp, and the finish line was closer than the start line. I got up and did the only thing I could do. I ran.

Pain was now my motivator, and after several more hours I spotted two people a few hundred yards ahead of me, collecting rope and signs from either side of the trail . . . the markers! I caught my fifteenth wind of the day, or so it seemed, and made a bolt towards them.

'Excuse me!' I said, wearily. 'Where am I?'

The two men looked slightly confused, like I'd just approached them and asked what year it was. One said, 'You're on Smeathes Ridge, about 10k from the finish. When did you start running?'

I realized there was no indication that I was officially involved in the event – I didn't have a race number, so I must have just looked like some chancer trying to join in a race he'd seen go past. Either way, I didn't care. I'd caught up with the markers, which meant I'd soon catch up with the back of the pack, and with 10k to go, not only did it look like I was going to reach the finish before anything was packed away, I might not even finish in last place!

I picked up the pace. My feet were in tatters but I had adapted my running style slightly to compensate for the pain. I felt a wave of emotion as I caught up with three people with race numbers attached to their tops. They looked like they were really struggling, and as I passed them I offered a few words of encouragement to help galvanize them for the final stretch. This is something I learned the real value of at mile 21 of the London Marathon, where my coach Charlie Dark's Run Dem Crew cheered me as I ran past with as much fanfare and gusto as if I was Mo Farah. 'Cheer Dem' assemble at mile 21 every year, empowering and lifting the spirits of every single person that runs, or walks, the marathon.

The selfless, congratulatory nature of running is what made me truly fall in love with it. When you light a fire under someone in a way that inspires and emboldens them, it can help restore not just their energy but also their sense of worth. When you feel like people have your back and are desperate for you to achieve, that's powerful; and so, despite being on my absolute last legs, I made an effort to pull some heartening words from my fellow runners as we all approached the final stretch of the Ridgeway.

When the Avebury Stone Circle came into view I felt like crying. It's a very moving sight in itself, but it also signified that I was nearly at the end of the race. I'd passed a number of people in the final few kilometres, including, to their amazement, Team Heads Together, who I would now wait for at the end. As the finish line came into view I heard an excited voice coming through the tannoy:

'. . . and there he is! The man who started the race thirteen hours late is about to finish!'

I smiled. The organizers must have read my tweet after all. As I crossed the line I was greeted by smiles and high-fives and hugs from people I didn't know. I felt elated, tired and weary, and just so relieved to have finished the race. I'd run ninety-two kilometres in seventeen hours. Writing now, I can't fully comprehend it – there is absolutely no way I'd be able to do that again. Something about that day, about everything that led up to it and the belief I had in myself, it all came together.

Within the hour I was reunited with Team Heads Together, who were all very tired and happy and ready to go home. After charging my phone enough to get in touch with Mike, I went to collect my bag, then jumped in a minibus bound for London with the rest of the Heads Together crew. I hadn't decided in advance what to do after RTTS, but it was clear to me that I needed a couple of days' rest before I set off on the walk again.

14

After what felt like a long drive Sofia and the team dropped me off somewhere near Stratford early on Monday morning. The plan was to go and stay with my best friend Freeman for a couple of nights, rest up, then jump on a train back up to North Yorkshire on the Wednesday. I was pleased to see my mate and catch up, but I was so shattered after the race that only a few minutes after arriving at his place I was in bed and out like a light. I slept, as he does, deeper and sounder than a hibernating bear.

The following day the two of us hung out for a few hours before Freeman went to work. He ordered me to stay in bed, but by three o'clock my legs were beginning to get twitchy. I noticed on Instagram that my coach, Charlie, had posted that Run Dem Crew would be assembling in the basement of the Ace Hotel in Shoreditch in a few hours. I hadn't been there since the London Marathon medal ceremony, an annual event organized by Charlie to recognize the achievements and journeys of the crew members who ran the marathon. I'd got to know Charlie in a very one-on-one way during filming, but on the night of the medal ceremony I saw the side of him that his crew sees – and what an inspiring leader he is. Since Charlie founded Run Dem Crew in 2007 as an alternative to 'traditional' running clubs, the crew has grown to over five hundred runners.

The night of the medal ceremony was one of the most unexpectedly beautiful events I've ever been to. I didn't have a clue what I was walking into; all I knew was I had to write some feelings about running the London Marathon on a sheet of paper and bring it along with my medal. I recognized a few of the faces from the cheer zone at mile 21 and, just like at that moment in the race, I was greeted with a warmth and reverence I wasn't sure I deserved. But back then I knew nothing about the crew, or 'Crew Love', as Charlie kept referring to it; all I knew was that it had this covert, underground feeling, like a more positive and less violent version of *Fight Club*. After spending a night immersed in it and receiving my medal from my other coach and now good friend Chevy Rough, who co-hosted the medal ceremony with Charlie, I knew it wouldn't be the last time I'd see these people. I'd had no idea communities like this existed, especially in London – and especially just down the road from where I'd experienced the darkest and loneliest time in my life. The Run Dem Crew community began to change the way I viewed society, and ever since I'd got back on the road I'd felt myself trying to embolden the people I met, something I'd learned from Charlie and his crew.

Realizing I wouldn't get another chance before I finished my walk, I decided to head down to the Ace Hotel and join Run Dem Crew and tell my frankly ridiculous Race to the Stones story; I thought, of all people, they'd understand just how intense the experience was. I caught up with one or two of them then headed out for a light 10k with Baby Cheetahs. (RDC is so vast in numbers now that the crew divides into seven or eight groups every week so everyone can run with people who are at their level and pace.) I'm sure running coaches and people with common sense will be shaking their heads at the idea of me running 10k two days after running 100k, and they'd probably be right – it's not a great idea to put your body through more stress after it's exceeded its yearly dose in seventeen hours, but in terms of recovery – the mileage I was doing every day during the walk – it didn't feel like a bad thing to me.

The following day I got on a train and made the long journey north to Skipton, where I'd got my first lift down to the Chilterns. It always gave me such mixed feelings, travelling back to where I'd left off on public transport. It was weird to think about everything that had occurred in the weeks and months it had taken me to walk across the country – the people I'd met, the situations I'd ended up in, the places I'd seen – and then travel the same distance in just an hour or two.

When I got to Skipton it was about 4 p.m. There wasn't much time to find my stride so I walked north out of town via the very steep Park Hill, wandered slowly until I joined the Dales High Way, following the old stone walls that divide the fields and the raggedy sheep within them, and after seven or eight miles stopped a few miles short of Hetton and found a quiet spot to camp.

The Yorkshire Dales are, in my opinion, one of the more underrated and overlooked national parks in Britain. In its most southerly section, the Craven district, huge boulders of limestone of varying shapes and sizes pepper the green landscape in a way so unique to that area. It feels prehistoric, like the land has looked that way since the dawn of time.

I spent the morning and most of the afternoon of the next day in the Toad, hiding from the rain. I arrived in Hetton at around 6 p.m. and stumbled upon a beautiful country pub, the George Inn, which looked like it had been in the square for hundreds of years, slowly amassing a thick cloak of ivy that engulfed the stone outer walls. It looked so inviting I decided to treat myself to a proper dinner and perhaps some light, frothy conversation with the locals, as was becoming customary.

The inside of the pub was as rustic as I'd hoped it would

be. The fire roared from a brick fireplace covered in soot, and thick, crooked oak beams ran the length of the ceiling. On the walls were several framed watercolour paintings of what looked like Malham Cove, an incredible limestone formation that was only a few miles away. After an hour of chill time I remembered I'd yet to find a place to camp. I packed my things up and headed back out into the square, where I immediately fell in with a small group of raucous, twenty-something locals, who happened to be walking the same way as me. Their energy, slightly impudent as it was in the quiet village, drew me in. I introduced myself to them with more confidence than I can ever remember having and, after some fairly textbook pleasantries, was invited back to the cottage where they were having a party and where they said I was welcome to spend the night. It was there that I first met Molly.

Of all the things you go through that can have a negative effect on mental health, love has got to be one of the least talked about. Don't get me wrong, connecting with somebody and falling in love and having them love you back is one of the greatest things that can happen to a person, but I believe, in more cases than is comfortable to guess, it can also be one of the worst. Being in love can be the warmest and most content you'll ever feel, but it can also make you sick with worry – constantly questioning your worth, obsessing about what the other person is thinking or if they love you the same amount back, becoming paranoid to the point of torture that they'll find someone better than you ... Your mind can become a runaway train of delusion, self-criticism and jealousy before you even get to properly know the person you've fallen for.

I've been in enough relationships to know that your perception of a significant other can become distorted if you pin all your potential for happiness on them. That invariably makes what should be a beautiful situation – two human beings connected by a shared feeling of deep attraction – feel stilted and stressful. I'm not saying the full span of a relationship can be compromised by such feelings (although I dare say one or two might go that far), but I'm pretty confident that every relationship will have to endure someone feeling like this at some point. And it's hard to deal with. *Really* fucking hard.

The thing is, you can't apply logic to love because it's about the closest thing we get to experiencing real magic in this life. Attraction and feelings of deep caring for an individual spring up on you without warning and with little consideration for what else is happening in your life and your mind at that time, and when a connection happens when you feel it really shouldn't it can mess with your head worse than anything.

We headed along a row of beautiful, old stone cottages, and it turned out that the one at the end was our destination. I tried desperately to keep the five-out-of-ten conversation I had initiated with the group going. They didn't have any idea who I was, and walking along in silence was the absolute last thing I should be doing if I wanted to be made to feel welcome. Without knowing how else to break the ice, I chucked on the broken record again and started telling the story of the walk. After a brief sum-up of my route, laced with a few wry anecdotes about people I'd met along the way, it felt like I'd said enough for everyone to feel quite chuffed I was there, so I was free to relax and start enjoying myself.

I found a seat by the fire in the small, cosy living room, and felt comfortable enough having a moment to myself to be still and observe the party. The warmth of the fire toasted my face and the sound of multiple conversations filled the house. It was the perfect balance between chilled and energetic.

A young woman came and sat next to me, and I turned to her and smiled.

'Someone just told me you're walking around the whole country,' she said. The light from the fire danced playfully in her eyes as she waited for me to speak. She was beautiful.

'That's right,' I said, gazing back at her.

'That's so fucking cool!'

I didn't know how to respond. In an instant, she'd become the centre of my focus and for a second or two I just froze.

'Er . . . what's your name?' I eventually said, fumbling.

'I'm Molly.'

'Jake,' I said.

Something stirred, a tingling warmth. I felt like I already knew this person, or maybe it was just a deep desire to want to know her.

This is the part of falling in love that's magical. I believe there's way more to life on earth than we know. To explain attraction and connection, we have to assume there's a force we cannot feel and which light doesn't touch, but it's still very much there. There are inexplicable times when space just seems to vibrate and everything around us feels charged.

Molly and I sat there for hours, locked in deep conversation about my journey, about mental health and life in general. She was so easy to talk to, and I enjoyed listening to her. When I talked about my passion for adventure and new experiences her eyes burned brighter than the fire in front of her. I sensed that it was the type of inspiration she really needed. My own thoughts, however, were far less together than our conversation suggested. Between every new topic, in every moment of silence, my eyes wandered from her eyes down to her mouth as my desire for her grew stronger.

After a few hours, most people had started to leave or disperse around the cottage and its garden, and there were now only a few stragglers left, engrossed in late-night heart-to-hearts. Molly had gone a little quiet and stared pensively into the dying embers of the fire, her eyes calm but alive like moonlit pools. There was a brief silence and, realizing I might be staring at her, I turned my gaze away and followed her eye line towards the fire. In that moment, as abruptly as a cough or a sneeze, she blurted out a crushing piece of information.

'I have a boyfriend.'

Shit.

The timing threw me, but it was an understandable thing to mention – I mean, I hadn't asked her if she had a boyfriend, nor had I braved leaning in at any point, but she clearly felt this was the time to clear that up.

'Oh,' I said.

For the first time since we'd started talking there was an awkwardness. We were both, however, very drunk by this point, and did our best to move on in a way that only two very drunk people can: we switched up the conversation and pretended like nothing weird had happened. Which worked fine, I guess, for a bit.

As the last embers died our conversation moved on to family. Molly told me something deeply personal, which I, having been through something similar, was able to understand in a way that seemed to touch her deeply. Our eyes met in quiet solemnity, and the two of us just sat and stared at one another. *Space vibrating.* Our hands touched. I felt sure that something was about to happen, and there was no stopping it. She blinked nervously and took a deep breath.

'Are you staying here tonight?' she asked.

My heart skipped a beat. I stared back at her for a second. There was no one else left in the room.

'Yes,' I said.

Slowly, we stood up, our fingers clasped together, and climbed the stairs. As we walked it felt like there were a billion tiny explosions orbiting in the air all around us, and when we reached the room where I'd left my things, I let go of her hand and quietly opened the door. Molly let out a nervous breath before walking in, almost like she was allowing her body to do what her mind knew she shouldn't. I hesitated for a second then followed her, closing the door behind me. Inside, we stared at each other for a moment. Molly looked scared. It just didn't feel right. She closed her eyes and leaned her head towards mine. I gulped. Our lips touched and for the briefest of moments a wave of pleasure relaxed both our bodies. My shoulders dropped as I closed my eyes and reached my hand out to touch her face. But I didn't make it. Molly snapped her body back and put her head in her hands.

'I can't,' she said, shaking her head.

I looked away. I didn't want her to feel my eyes on her as she wrestled with herself. From not being able to break eye contact, the two of us could no longer hold each other's eyes for longer than a second. I desperately wanted her to stay with me, but deep down we both knew that couldn't happen. I felt I had to put the brakes on. It was clear she'd regret what would happen if either of us gave in to our urges, so after a forced jump back into rationality, the equivalent of a cold shower, I guess, Molly crept out, leaving me disappointed and alone, but kind of sure that we'd done the right thing.

I woke to the smell of bacon a few hours later and some muted chatter coming from downstairs. My room was lit up with a soft glow that suggested an overcast morning sky. After a few minutes of stretching and snorting I got dressed and headed down to join the others.

They were sat in the garden, and in the daylight I was able to take a proper look at my surroundings. In the distance I could just make out the limestone bridge that passed over the stream and, from what I remembered from looking at the map the day before, led to Malham Cove, a few miles or so north of the village. It looked so classically English, like a location for a period drama.

I looked around for Molly, but I couldn't see her. I wondered if she had actually ended up staying over – she'd mentioned that she lived really close by. Some genius had bought a load of bacon and sausages and was pouring out mugs of tea for everyone. An absolute masterstroke, I thought, as I looked around at what could easily have been a low-spirited morning after. Having been treated to a sausage sandwich with brown sauce, accompanied by ten minutes of profoundly bland conversation with a guy whose breath smelt like ten different drinks all at once, I felt some puzzled looks coming my way. It appeared they were struggling to remember who the fuck I was.

I decided it was probably time to leave. I darted back to the room where I'd slept, packed up my things, hoisted everything on to my back and waved a quiet, insecure goodbye through to the group in the garden, avoiding the detritus of empty cans and bottles strewn about. But as I walked through the front room, I found a second huddle of people. The conversation looked sincere, with everyone leaning in, listening intently to the person who was talking and looking, as beautiful as she was, decidedly uneasy. *Molly*. Inevitably she saw me and I motioned that I was leaving. She came out to the front of the house with me, her arms folded in a self-comforting hug. I could see now just how beautiful she was. Her eyes, so striking, alert and watchful, sparkled as if the embers of the fire had somehow become trapped inside. Her red hair

fell to her shoulders, a few untamed flyaways breaking free
to rest elegantly across her face.

To my relief, she looked genuinely happy to see me.

'Morning,' I said.

'Morning.'

'Did you sleep OK?'

'Not too bad,' she said. 'You?'

'Not bad.'

We stared at each other for a lingering moment. 'Sorry I
can't stick around, I've got a lot of walking to do today and if
I don't go soon the hangover won't let me,' I said.

Molly nodded, then stepped forward and put her arms
around me. She smelt amazing, like nice shampoo with a
hint of burnt coal from sitting so close to the fireplace, and
I held her for one last moment, feeling her completely, before
letting go.

'See you then,' she said.

'Yeah, bye,' I said.

It didn't feel right leaving, but there was no reason to stay,
and definitely no point in asking if she wanted to come with
me (as desperately as I wanted to). As I turned to walk away
I got a horrible feeling, like I was at that exact moment missing a chance to grasp something really special. There was a
part of me that thought I might find 'the one' on my walk
around Britain – not in a genuine way, more in a romantic
love story way – and just then it felt like Molly could have
been that person. I hesitated for a second, my back to her,
then without looking back made my way down the road and
out of Hetton.

Over the next few days I passed through the numerous fells
and valleys that make up this glorious section of the Pennine
Way. The view from Pen-y-ghent is exquisite and as I looked

out I couldn't help but think about my journey, about what it all meant. I'd had a succession of hugely profound moments over the previous year, and they were now all beginning to feel connected, like one couldn't have happened without another. For the first time I considered that perhaps I wasn't in control of it all, as I'd thought I was, that maybe there was something else guiding me, something non-physical, maybe even transcendental. I looked back at everything that had happened to me on the walk, looking for evidence of this guiding hand – the chance encounters that led to what I considered to be big, life-altering realizations about myself and about the world, realizations that I felt had changed my mindset and facilitated what I considered to be unimaginably demanding physical achievements. I had thought before that this walk was bigger than me in some way, that it might have less to do with the challenge itself and more to do with the effect it was having on me, and other people through me, but as I traversed the villages, fields and ridges of the Pennine Way I noticed that from having blissfully accepted that everything felt right and made complete sense, my perspective had switched, and I now felt that I understood so little of the what, how and why of everything happening in the way it was.

Molly stayed in my thoughts for days. As fleeting as it was, our meeting had flicked yet another switch, and although all the signs were pointing to it being little more than a romantic ships-passing-in-the-night situation, my gut was telling me there was something more profound about our meeting. We hadn't exchanged numbers and I didn't know her surname, so there was no way of making contact, but I got a sense that we'd meet again. Somehow, this wasn't the end, and as the days rolled on with nothing to distract me from my thoughts I began to believe that there was something fateful about the night we met.

A feeling of loneliness crept in for the first time in almost eight months of walking solo, and it hit me with such force I couldn't escape it. Meeting Molly had made me realize that, after being on my own for so many years, I was ready to let someone into my life again. What made it harder was that I missed her, such a strange thing to feel after spending just one evening with someone.

I spent two days walking the twenty-three miles of the Pennine Way to Hawes, then changed course and took the main road west for a further twenty-five miles, leaving York-shire and heading towards the Lake District town of Kendal. I had mixed feelings about leaving Yorkshire; it was a county that had been welcoming, neighbourly and fun, as its reputation suggested it might be, but it had also been where I'd begun to deconstruct the walk in new and slightly confusing ways. My mood had been affected as a result and without anything other than the walk to distract them, my thoughts were spiralling. I even found myself, on some occasions, oblivious to the scenery, which was unbelievable, as the Yorkshire Dales are right up there with some of the most impressive landscapes in England. It's only there that you find the colours and gradients of a moorland riddled with limestone, and when I ceased ruminating enough to stop and properly take it in I remembered how lucky I was to be able to experience the country in this way. I'd never been especially proud of being English, not in a political, histori-cal sense anyway. But edging through the countryside mile by mile, you can't help but feel a deep sense of pride. With this in mind, I felt myself looking forward to seeing what the Lake District had to offer. The forecast was for a wet week, so I'd been on the lookout for someone to put me up for a night or two.

A week or so previously I'd been contacted by a woman called Isabel who'd offered me a stay at her house in Sedbergh. I spoke to her on the phone and, deciding that she sounded nice enough, gratefully accepted her invitation. She lived alone in a residential street about fifteen minutes' walk from the town centre. When I got there I was struck by how attractive she was. She had wavy blonde hair down to her shoulders, expressive eyes and a beautiful smile. We ate dinner in her back garden and in the late-afternoon light she looked almost heavenly, her eyes twinkling as she spoke to me. I found myself wondering if she'd invited me round because she liked the look of me too. We went inside her cosy wooden-floored house and after a spontaneous hug in the living room I leaned in and kissed her. She seemed shy at first, and for a moment I thought I'd misread the situation, but a few minutes later we were kissing passionately, bumping into the table and the bookcase, working our way over to the sofa. It felt incredible to be intimate with someone, to feel someone's skin on mine, to be locked in such an intense physical embrace.

A passionate night followed, but when I woke the following morning I felt guilty. I could sense that I'd transferred my longing for Molly on to Isabel, and that was a really shitty thing to do. Not for the first time in my life, I put my own desires over the feelings of another human being. I didn't like to think that maybe Isabel had feelings for me beyond the physical, and I'd got carried away, said misleading things, things I wished I could tell Molly. I'd treated Isabel like a brief love interest in the story of 'me'; blinded by lust and a desire for intimacy, I'd shown her none of the respect she deserved for inviting me into her home.

Isabel letting me into her house was far riskier and took far more trust than if it was the other way round, and to behave the way I did after she'd invited me in is something I'm deeply ashamed of. But what happened happened, and there was nothing I could do to take it back. I sent Isabel a message of apology some time after, but I never heard from her again.

15

I was beginning to feel a bit lost and confused, and now guilty, after a few of my recent encounters. Feeling like I could do with a distraction, I called my friend Kirk, who had been in touch a week or so ago to ask if he could join me once I reached Cumbria. When I asked him if there was a particular spot he was thinking of he told me he wanted to go to the northern fells and climb to the top of Blencathra mountain near Skiddaw. His dad, Graham, died in a helicopter crash when Kirk was thirteen and his ashes were scattered at a lake called Scales Tarn in a hollow on the side of Blencathra. When I asked why his family had chosen to scatter his dad's ashes halfway up a mountain, Kirk proudly told me that his old man used to enjoy abseiling and his favourite thing to do was to fasten his harness on backwards, climb to the top of Blencathra's notorious Sharp Edge ascent then run down the mountain face first. I told Kirk that I would climb Sharp Edge with him if he promised not to bring any abseiling gear and, on a thankfully very spontaneous whim, he dropped everything, borrowed a car and drove three hundred miles to come out and meet me.

Kirk and I had lived together in Brighton while I was shooting *Mind over Marathon*, my second spell living in that house, and after I'd left the landlord had sold the property and the new owner evicted everyone. Kirk, along with my other housemates, Jess, James and Lauren, was being kicked out, and our beautiful home, where we'd spent so many good years, was going to be turned into student accommodation.

They, along with everyone who had ever lived or enjoyed good times at Ditchling Rise over the years, were preparing one last blowout, an end-of-the-world party, and it happened to coincide with Kirk's trip up to the Lakes. We decided that Kirk would drive up to meet me, the two of us would spend a quality day in the Lake District and then I'd drive back down to Brighton with him for the party. I'd have to catch a coach back up to Kendal, but it didn't matter: making plans like this didn't feel like cheating anymore. The first few times I'd done it, I'd felt like I was in some way betraying the seriousness of the challenge, but this far in, the walk, while still very much a challenge, had become my life, and in the same way that, if I'd had a steady job and someone had invited me to an event I had to travel across the country to, I felt a break in my routine could provide me with a much-needed release valve – especially since I'd become fraught with guilt and longing and prone to slightly obsessive existential thoughts lately. No matter how much pleasure and exercise and soul-searching time I was gaining from walking around the country, the fact that it had become my new 'normal' meant that any stress I was experiencing was typically walk related, and to complete the thing without burning out along the way, like I burnt out while I was living in east London, it was crucial to give myself the occasional break.

Stepping away from stress feels really unnatural at first, almost like you're embracing failure, but being able to put some temporary distance between yourself and a situation that's causing you to feel overwhelmed isn't failure, it's a survival skill. Since my mental health reached Defcon 1 back in March 2016, I'd learned that stress is my body's way of telling me that it's under threat. In the months leading up to my final days in east London I was under a tremendous amount of work stress. My foggy state of mind, combined with my reckless lifestyle, meant I'd fallen behind on admin. Reports weren't being submitted on time, important documents weren't filed away properly; I was existing in a constant state of catch-up. My only thought was 'I can't take any time for myself until I've caught up with all of this,' which I now acknowledge was a huge mistake and one that I feel directly contributed to me becoming ill. I thought then that time away from work would result in me falling further behind, but I now think that, actually, if I'd taken a step back and focused on looking after me rather than worrying about work, I might have given myself a chance of being able to see what needed to be done and to organize myself and my time more effectively. Once we acknowledge that, it's up to us to gauge the level of threat and act accordingly. For example, if I'm feeling stressed out but I'm still able to manage tasks, work resolutely and find some joy in life, I gauge the threat as medium, meaning it's time for me to dig deeper, because proving to myself that I can stand up to the heat by powering through can be really beneficial to my self-esteem. If, however, I feel panicky, beleaguered or like I've lost control, then I know the threat is reaching critical and it's time to slow down, regroup and think about stepping away.

Imagine the feeling of stress, all that adrenaline and cortisol charging around your body, as an air-raid siren, telling you that a bomb's about to hit and it's time to find cover. We can probably agree that the correct decision is *not* to stand stubbornly and defiantly while bombs rain down around you, which means we should also agree that ducking for shelter until the planes have passed is not failure to deal with the situation. Acknowledging that you're not fully in control of your emotions means you're better equipped to decide how best to deal with the situation, and making a sensible choice at that point gives back some control.

Although the recent stuff with Molly and Isabel hadn't exactly got me to Defcon 1 level stress, it had affected me enough to make me realize that maybe an opportunity to briefly return home and spend a night with my friends wasn't to be wasted. I was clearly craving amity and human closeness, and who better to see to that than the people I really love?

Before that, though, Kirk and I had a couple of days in the Lake District. I found a dingy pub in the centre of Kendal with low ceilings, dark walls and busted light bulbs, and after going to the bar and ordering a tea I hid in a quiet nook near the back, got comfy in a musty booth and waited for him to arrive. I was there a good few hours, and spent the majority of them replaying the events of the last few days in my head and wishing I could get hold of Molly. *What's she doing right now?* I longed for her company, to find out more about who she is, and to feel the electricity I felt between us on the night we met. I even caught myself looking up the cost of a train to visit her, at which point I realized I needed to get a grip. I spent the next few hours reading my book, listening to podcasts – anything to distract me from thinking about her.

When Kirk finally walked through the door, hair wet from the rain and looking very tasty in his yellow raincoat (clothes always look great on Kirk), I noticed he looked a little drained and fed up after the drive, so I suggested grabbing a drink and hanging out for an hour before heading off. Over a couple of swift halves of very cheap, very murky real ale, Kirk told me that before he left Brighton he had taken the liberty of booking us a cabin for the night at the White Horse, a pub and bunkhouse just off the main road at the foot of Blencathra, thirty-odd miles away. I'd been so distracted I hadn't even thought about sleeping arrangements, probably assuming that we would simply two's up in the Toad; which knowing Kirk as well as I do, is an idea that would have flown about as far as he could throw me.

Kirk and I met in Brighton in the spring of 2010 through a mutual friend, Paul, while Paul and I were recruiting for a new band. Kirk was drumming for another Brighton band called Trippin' Violet at the time, and was sold to me as a drummer 'like Tommy Lee' of Mötley Crüe, which, after a couple of practice sessions with him, I decided was actually a pretty great description.

Covered in tattoos and painfully good-looking, Kirk definitely had a presence, and after those practice sessions it was clear he wasn't just a handsome face but also a very tight, very loud drummer – just what we were after. After recruiting Dan (my old friend from Maldon who put me up in Southampton when the walk first began) on bass, and another mutual friend, AJ, on second guitar, the five of us formed Deadband, a very fast, very loud punk-rock outfit that, sadly, turned into one of those landfill bands that never made it out of the rehearsal studio.

The reason we never played a gig was because, despite initially writing a handful of genuinely great songs, we always practised at Studio 284, a grungy squat-like rehearsal space under the road arches in Brighton which we loved because the owner let us drink and smoke and stay as long as we wanted so long as we locked up when we left. This inevitably turned every practice into a heavy drinking session, where we'd end up playing one of our songs over and over again because it 'just sounds so fucking good'.

Kirk and I quickly became close friends. He was the only person I asked if he fancied coming along with me when I decided to walk around Britain, and although at the time of asking he couldn't quite get a handle on the idea, on account of being 'unbelievably high' at the time, I was really pleased that he'd now come to join me for a portion of my journey.

After we finished our pints it was starting to get dark, so we set off, driving north on the A6 towards Keswick. At first, everything was great. Kirk had queued up an album by one of our favourite bands, The Bronx, which we dutifully sang and air-drummed along to on the drive, as was tradition; and everything was going great until after a few miles Kirk noticed the engine was getting hot. He'd borrowed our housemate Jess's car and so knew nothing about what condition it was in. In an obvious bid not to kill the buzz, Kirk vowed to 'just keep an eye on it', rather than address the fact that the car had no breakdown cover and that if anything went wrong we could end up in quite serious trouble.

Unfortunately, as we were in the Lake District, the route involved a bit of uphill driving, which in turn meant a lot of revs on the engine, and after fifteen minutes or so the dashboard lit up like a fruit machine. Almost immediately, the time for pretending was over; the time to start worrying was now upon us. After reaching the crest of a particularly steep hill Kirk suggested we stop to give the engine a minute to cool down. We pulled over and turned the engine off, at which point we felt the full force of the wind on all sides of us; it had picked up significantly since we'd left Kendal. Above the distant horizon the sky was a deep, almost royal blue on one side of us and absolutely jet black on the other, and the land ahead was so dark it was basically invisible. Realizing how cut off we were, Kirk's attention was momentarily diverted away from the overheated engine, and he said, with no discernible irony: 'This sort of place is only good for two things – burying bodies . . . and dogging.'

Theatrical as it sounded, there was some truth to that; we were in the arse end of nowhere with a cooked engine and no breakdown cover, and all of a sudden the possibility of being marooned there at the top of that hill was becoming unnervingly real.

'Right, bonnet up,' said Kirk, springing into action. For some reason I was always forgetting how into cars and engines he is. Whenever we or someone we know has had car trouble in the past, he's always seemed to know all the right words and what needs doing, meaning that of all the possible friends to be in a situation like this with, Kirk was actually the guy I'd want.

'Radiator's bone dry,' he announced indisputably, furiously rubbing his hands together. I could feel how cold it was outside on him.

'What do we do?' I asked sheepishly, praying that by some miracle he had a spare water tank in the boot or something.

'Dunno, mate,' he said, truthfully.

One of Kirk's best (and sometimes worst) qualities is his complete, occasionally very harsh honesty. He doesn't go out of his way to be cruel, but if you want the truth you're always guaranteed it with him, because he's one of the few people I know who doesn't (and doesn't just say he doesn't) give one shit what anyone thinks of him. It's the thing that's probably the most polarizing about us, and a part of his personality I've always admired. I often find myself thinking how much easier life would be if I was relieved of the constant feeling that I've somehow offended or upset people, or made them angry, or made their life difficult in some way. In my mind, where anxieties about my interpersonal relationships rain down more or less constantly, guilt hangs over me like a funnel, collecting them all and drenching me in them. I worry about how people feel about me so much sometimes that I consciously don't speak to friends for a while to see if *they* get in touch with *me*. If they don't, and my worst suspicion/fear

(I'm never quite sure which it is) is confirmed, it isn't uncommon for me to jump to the conclusion that that person simply doesn't like me anymore, and instead of getting annoyed about it, as some people seem to, it gets internalized and feeds my inner self-loathing beast. I feel kind of embarrassed admitting this. It feels needy and histrionic to put it into words and read it back, and it's not a part of my character I'm particularly stoked about putting out there. However, I do have a way of coping with it that I believe could be of some value to someone – perhaps you – who hasn't got past the very painful and damaging internalizing stage yet.

So, when I become worried about what people think of me, here's three things I do.

1. I make myself feel better about *me*. When I look in the mirror and hate who I see, I feel like that's the person everyone else sees too. When I start treating myself with some respect and focus on making myself feel healthy and responsible, I not only start to like who I see when I look in the mirror, I start to care a lot less about what people see when they look at me. To like who I see, I: run, eat well, brush my teeth properly, wear clean clothes, make my bed every morning, wake up early, keep my personal space tidy, do press-ups, take vitamins, respond to emails, get a grip on my finances, run again, etc., etc. This might seem like the most clichéd self-help list of all time, but doing these types of things daily does genuinely make me care less what people think of me.

2. I remind myself that everyone is probably like me. It really helps to be conscious that everyone: wakes up, remembers things they have to do, doesn't do

them, eats breakfast, shits breakfast, doesn't drink enough water, worries about money, fears that they don't talk to their family enough, remembers things they're embarrassed about, looks at the same face in the mirror every day, scrolls mindlessly on their phone, does a big shop, loses their belongings, wishes they looked different, pretends not to be bothered about things when they are, feels judged, compares themselves to others, has a weird thing on their body they're too afraid to get checked out, abides by laws they had no say in deciding, desires someone they can't have, gets too tired to do any-thing, and then goes to bed. The amount of shit we all carry around with us every day is back-breakingly heavy, and on days when I can really feel the weight, my wish to engage with someone – anyone – trying to have a frothy, droll conversation with me is usually somewhere around the 'nil' mark. To be mindful of that is to be more understanding of everyone else's situation. Everyone *is* you; they're just having a different type of hard, busy life.

3. I do my best to maintain the relationships that matter. This one is slightly more nuanced than the first two, and there are a couple of things I always have to bear in mind. Key number one is to not be too hard on myself for not being able to do it. Let me quickly draw your attention to the 'do my best' part of the opening sentence. If I'm truly honest with myself about doing my best to stay in touch with people (which includes not using energy if I don't have any to do so), then I recognize that everyone else has to be in the same boat, which means my instinct is to sympathize with people rather than

hold them responsible for making me feel unwanted. The second key is to absolutely, categorically, avoid 'keeping score'. If I'm trying harder to stay in touch with someone (who you know is a true friend and not someone who you just like) who's not reciprocating the amount of effort I'm putting in, I have to be OK with that. The bottom line is, if we're talking, it's good; we're maintaining what we have. If someone seems to be assuming you'll be their friend regardless of how little effort they put in, all that means is they think and behave differently to you – and of *course* they do. They: have different parents, have different genes, were born at a different time, have been places you've never been, developed loves and fears differently, have been humiliated differently, just can't deal with people sometimes, are interested in topics you aren't, have different circadian rhythms, work in a different job, were brought up with a different set of values, changed a little every time someone close to them died, deal with different people to you every day, etc., etc.

A true friend shouldn't put pressure on another to fit into their archetype of what a 'true friend' is. Putting pressure on people leads to resentment, so the trick is to give up on the idea that other people's behaviour is a variable you can control – because it just isn't. The only thing you can control is your reaction, and the way that I've learned to control my reactions is to (in the least grumpy way I can) never expect anything from anybody. I've spent a long time and tried really hard to implement this, and as a result I'd truthfully say that I've become more independent, I resent people less and I'm pleasantly surprised and grateful whenever a friend does something for me. So I'm sold on it.

Remember, people's behaviour is not a reflection of you, and when a friend behaves differently to you (including how much of their time they choose to give you) that does not necessarily mean they are complacent, or they don't care.

Be understanding. Be empathetic. Be honest. That's how you maintain friendship.

Kirk and I had been sitting by the side of the road, unsure what to do, for about five minutes. We desperately needed to fill up the water tank but we couldn't remember passing any garages on the way and there was nothing to suggest there were any ahead of us either. The wind outside was howling wildly and the rain had turned into hail, rapping incessantly against the roof of the car like thousands of tiny pick-axes. A light from behind us shone through the interior, lighting up the dash. A van pulled up alongside us. It was the police. Kirk wound his window down, and we were once again slapped with a shrill, polar wind and, this time, the odd shard of icy shrapnel.

'Everything all right?' asked one of the officers. With those round vowel sounds so typical of the accent in the north-west making everyone sound so safe and well-intentioned, the law enforcement there are probably contenders for the least threatening-sounding police in Britain. It could easily have been Peter Kay or Mrs Merton pulling up alongside us.

'Our radiator's too hot,' said Kirk good-naturedly, presumably influenced by the officer's accent. 'I don't suppose you boys have some water, do you?'

There was a pause, and the look on the officer's face suggested Kirk's slightly cheeky use of the word 'boys' hadn't gone down too well. 'Nope,' he replied, unhelpfully.

Another pause. It was beginning to get awkward. The hail was coming down even more heavily now, and the officer wound his window up so that just his eyes were showing.

'OK, well, do you know where the nearest garage is?' said Kirk, his tone a little sterner than before.

'There's nothing ahead for about ten miles, sir.' His accent was no longer endearing, and all I could focus on was his manner, which was kind of annoying. I noticed Kirk's left hand grip the steering wheel harder.

'Fancy going to get us some water?' he said. I stifled a smile. Kirk is excellent at subtle confrontation, another thing I admire about him.

'Nope,' came the reply again. He was not the least bit amused.

I was a bit perplexed by how quickly things had escalated.

'You should move on. It isn't safe to be parked here,' the policeman said at last and, just like that, the van pulled away, leaving Kirk and I alone by the roadside.

'Well, thanks a bunch, dickhead,' said Kirk, staring in disbelief. He spent the next few minutes venting, mostly about police and there being no water in the radiator and us needing a 'fucking miracle' to get out of the mess we were in.

While he was carrying on I had a thought. *There might not be a garage, but that doesn't mean there's no water.* I took my phone out and opened the OS app. I followed the road ahead until my finger came to what looked like a small river or canal which, at first glance, seemed to run underneath the road. I'd lost my aluminium water bottles at some point during the Race to the Stones saga, but did have a one-litre plastic bottle I'd been refilling continuously over the past couple of weeks. I reached back and heaved it from the side pocket of my pack.

'I think I have a plan. Look, there's a stream a mile or so down the road,' I said, trying to curb the immeasurable satisfaction I was deriving from this, frankly, genius idea. 'We're at the top of this hill now, right? So it should be down-hill the whole way there. D'you reckon we can make it?'

Kirk shrugged, a little too indifferently for my liking, then fidgeted back into his seat and reached for the ignition. The plan was useless if we couldn't get down there and we held our breath as he turned the key and started the engine. For a moment we sat perfectly still, listening to the car purr like a grumpy old cat we were trying not to wake. After a few sec-onds, Kirk, as delicately as I'd ever seen him touch anything, released the handbrake and exhaled through pursed lips as we pulled away and rolled into the darkness.

'So far, so-so,' he said after a few seconds, his hands firmly in the ten-to-two position. He was driving so gingerly I had to stifle a slightly nervous laugh.

Some mirth, thankfully, was just what was needed to break the ice and as we trundled downhill the two of us burst into giggles and broke into an ironic acappella version of Steppenwolf's 'Born to be Wild'. Even though we were, in all probability, plunging head first into an ordeal, at least we could see the funny side, which meant that, as bad as the situation could potentially get, being together was going to make the whole thing more bearable.

After a minute or so we'd picked up enough speed for Kirk to stop revving and for the car to just roll. Fearing we might overheat again, he cut the engine, his know-how com-ing into play, and we coasted down the hill. He looked slightly panicked when he noticed that the steering was 'getting heavy', the breaks were 'getting squishy' and the headlights were 'dim as fuck'. Thankfully, the hail storm had passed and the wind appeared less violent now that we weren't at the crest of a hill, so as we rolled we were treated to a few moments of calm as we prepared to enter survival mode.

'Right, where's this river, then?'

'It should be coming up any second now,' I said, watching our position on the app's GPS edge closer and closer to the thin blue line that had 'Wasdale Beck' written over it (I wasn't sure, so I was silently praying it *was* a river). It was now some fifty yards ahead of us.

'Well, keep your eyes peeled, because I may as well be driving through a swamp at the moment.'

The hills on the horizon sat calmly, like motionless black waves. Every now and then the clouds ahead parted and the moon cast just enough light to brighten the road. As we approached what looked like a bridge I noticed the moonlight shimmering wildly off the land on my side.

'There!' I shouted excitedly, and Kirk heaved the car over to the side of the road. We flung the doors open and raced to take a look. Cascading underneath us was a canalized section of a, as Kirk put it cheerily, 'fully flowing, angry fucking river'. We leapt into action. I pegged it back to the car and grabbed my bottle, and when I got back Kirk had already bunked over a ramshackle old fence and was teetering on what looked like rocks on the banks of the water. I clambered down to join him and shimmied further down so I could get right next to the water. It was moving so fast and, as it splashed on to my face and hands, I could feel it was ice cold.

When I got close enough I bent down and, gripping it tightly, lowered my bottle into the drink and filled it. Then we scrambled back up the rocks, over the fence and to the car. Kirk popped the bonnet and joined me at the engine just as I began pouring. The speed and the excitement we were operating at, it was like we'd found gold in that river, and as the last of the water went in we cheered jubilantly.

'What's that?' Kirk said, hushing down our celebrations.

'What's what?'

'Shhh.'

Kirk squatted down in front of the car and I heard a faint trickle coming from below us.

'No,' I said, my gut flipping as I realized what it was. To our horror, the level of water in the tank was now half what it had been a few moments before.

'It's pissing out the bottom,' said Kirk, in a tone that said, unmistakably, *We're fucked*.

At the base of the water tank was a small hole. Anything we put in was going to come straight out the bottom, and with nothing to doctor the hole with, it was clear we were now in an actual, categorically bad 'situation'. There was only one thing we could do.

Over the next five or ten minutes I ran down to the river, filled the bottle, ran back up to the fence and passed it to Kirk; Kirk ran to the car, dumped the water in the tank, then ran down to the fence and threw it – *Carefully!* – to me. Again and again, until the tank was full. Then we jumped in the car and got going as fast as we could. If there hadn't been so much at stake, it might have been quite fun, but with our safety on the line it felt more like a deadly serious military operation.

We had literally no time to waste; all we could focus on was the fact that the water would have already started trickling out and it wouldn't be long before the engine overheated again. We drove the few miles to the end of the road without any trouble, but we were now about to join the M6, one of, if not the, busiest motorways in England. Luckily, it was late, and there weren't many cars on the road but, even so, pulling on to a motorway when there's a high chance of your vehicle conking out is a terrifying prospect. We tried not to think about that too much and held our breath, knowing that if we could just get to Penrith, which was thankfully only a few miles away, at least we'd be able to turn off and break down somewhere less dangerous.

We entered into what felt like a long period of silent prayer as we drove. Neither of us said a word. It was as if, if we maintained a state of 'pause', so would the level in the water tank. Desperate times were calling for desperately wishful measures, and it seemed to be working for a few minutes, right until the lights on the dash lit up and Kirk's hands once again gripped tight on the steering wheel.

'Shit.'

None of it was funny anymore. We were driving along the M6, a long way from home, with no breakdown cover, it was late, and if for any reason we had to stop the engine was going to die. Not a minute too soon our turn-off came into view and, as Kirk flicked on the indicator, we shared the briefest sense of relief as we prepared to come off the motorway. Ahead of us, as we descended towards a roundabout, we saw traffic lights. And they were red. We trundled towards them in what felt like slow motion, both of us desperately willing them to turn green. I realized that this was probably it – the end of the road. And as the car ground to a halt right in front of the roundabout, dashboard lights cutting out, engine letting out its final breath, the car died, and there it was. The end of the line. We were fucked.

We got out, pushed the car to the side of the road and stood there in silence for a while, not quite knowing what to say to each other. Our victory at the river had been short-lived and, with no cars on the road, Kirk began the tedious process of calling around Britain's main breakdown services, and all of them said, as predicted, that collecting us was going to cost a bomb, and even if we decided to shell out all they'd do was cart the car back to Brighton. After twenty minutes or so, Kirk, in a state of nervous desperation, I guess, even called his mum. It wasn't going to get us anywhere, but I understood why he did it. Sometimes it's just good to hear your mum's voice.

After half an hour or so, having completely lost hope, I noticed a pickup truck turn off the M6 and make its way down towards the roundabout. As it pulled up alongside us a man, possibly in his early thirties, pulled down the window and leaned across.

'Shit,' said the man.

'Yeah,' I said. It was an exchange that said all there was to say.

'Anything I can do?' He sounded like he genuinely wanted to help.

'Not unless you've got a couple of gallons of water knocking about,' said Kirk despairingly. 'Our radiator's packed up.'

'Say no more,' replied the man, and with that he wound his window up and drove away, turning sharply off the roundabout and heading down the A66 into the night.

Ten minutes passed, then fifteen. The temperature had dropped considerably and I was beginning to feel cold and tired, and as a result, headachey and nauseous. After twenty-five minutes I noticed a light in the distance and made out what looked to be a set of headlights buried in the black of the horizon coming up the A66 towards us. In the entire time we had been marooned, no other cars had passed, and I pushed my face hard against the inside of my coat until I could taste the zip, begging to something, anything, that it was our guy returning. As the headlights got closer I was able to make out the vehicle. It was the pickup – our man *had* returned – and as he got on to the roundabout and heroically looped around to meet us I felt such a thrill he might as well have been driving a chariot doing a victory loop at a Roman amphitheatre. I could see through the open passenger-side window that he'd brought with him an enormous – maybe ten-gallon – jerry can.

''Ere, you can have this,' he said cheerily. 'It's only about half full, but it should get you some of the way, eh?'

I felt a surge of relief as intense as anything I'd ever felt. I couldn't think of words big enough to thank him. He had saved us, truly. We did our best to express how pathetically grateful we were, and as he was about to drive away Kirk called out to him: 'Mate, what's your name?'

The man shot us both a mischievous grin and, in a tone so genuine and carefree, simply said: 'Why?'

Something about him reminded me of Alan, the recovering heroin addict who'd picked me up while I was hitchhiking down to Race to the Stones. Something made me wonder if he too was in some kind of recovery, and seizing the opportunities that came his way to right the wrongs in his past. He didn't seem to weigh up if he had the time, or if Kirk and I deserved his help; he just went and got us some water, no questions asked.

We'd been shivering by the side of the road for well over an hour by this point, so we lost no time filling the radiator and jumping in the car. As the car spluttered into life, we didn't even allow ourselves a moment to feel relieved. We still had eight or nine miles left to drive until we were safely out of the woods, and we weren't sure if the three or four gallons in the jerry can would be enough to get us the whole way. It was now midnight. We stopped at a lay-by and checked the water level. It was dropping, but we still had a bit of time before it was empty. We decided that, instead of letting the engine overheat, we'd pull into *every* lay-by to top the water up.

This turned out to be a blinding course of action. There were places to pull over every couple of minutes, and soon the two of us were like a well-oiled Formula 1 pit crew: buckles off, bottle cap off, door open, bonnet popped, water in, back on the road. We had it nailed all the way to the White Horse, and after we pulled into the car park and clambered out of the car, we shared a brief, comforting glance. The ordeal was over. We had made it.

The following morning we got up and left the bunkhouse early. We headed over to a stony track at the base of Blencathra and I was hit by all the refreshing smells of morning – damp grass, fresh air and a hint of wet tarmac – we still weren't too far from the main road. Within an hour we'd flanked the mountain's south side and were heading up a steep track on the lower slope of the fell. It was tough on our legs at first but after twenty minutes or so the incline eased off and we found ourselves walking along a long, level pathway deep in a valley that stretched far into the distance. The Lake District was given National Heritage status some years back, and it's so easy to see why. The vast, open landscape looks timeless, like it hasn't changed at all since the Earth was formed. Thinking what a privilege it was to be up there, I got momentarily caught up in 'What does it all mean?' thoughts. Would we be up there at all if I hadn't needed a distraction from feeling guilty about what had happened with Isabel?

Kirk snapped me out of it and drew my attention to Sharp Edge, emerging out of the fog half a kilometre or so north. I have to say it didn't look like much from a distance, but as we got closer the steepness of the ascent became clear and, forty minutes or so later, after a quiet moment at Scales Tarn for Kirk to remember his dad, the two of us got focused, strapped our backpacks on tight and began to climb. At that point, the only mountains I'd climbed since my walk began were Pen ỳ Fan and Mount Snowdon and, while they weren't exactly a run to the shops, the routes I'd taken hadn't posed any sort of real danger. Sharp Edge would be the first time scaling a mountain had the potential to go wrong, and as the last of the track disappeared we had to start choosing which of the small ledges looked safest to stand on.

The option to turn back soon evaporated and we were left with no option but to continue to the top. After ten minutes we reached a section known as the 'bad step', where many of the fatalities on the ascent had happened over the years. It's a deep crack in a section of the rock that is noticeably smoother and thus more slippery than the rest of Sharp Edge. Thankfully, despite some residual morning dew, it had been a dry start to the day, and so with patience and care, and Kirk reiterating his principle rule for the day – 'Don't fall' – we made it over the drop and were soon enough scrambling confidently towards the summit.

The wind thrashed us mercilessly as we reached the mountain top, marvelling at the miles of dark grey and green all around us. After some debriefing and admissions of how scared we'd been jumping over the 'bad step', we began our descent along the slightly longer but far easier walkers' track, and an hour or so later we were back in the White Horse, drinking hot chocolate and feeling like we'd accomplished more before breakfast than we had in the whole six months we'd lived together in Brighton.

Now we had to find somewhere, or someone, to fix the radiator so we could get back for the Ditchling Rise farewell party. We asked the landlord of the pub if he knew anyone; we'd managed to establish quite a good rapport with him after amusing him with a bouncy and self-deprecating account of our disastrous drive up. He made a couple of calls and within two hours we had left the car in the hands of Sid, a very capable-looking mechanic who after some friendly negotiation agreed to fit a new water tank for a very reasonable price.

The drive down to Brighton was blissfully painless and we arrived to find the party in full swing. That house in Ditchling Rise had acted as a social hub for so many of my friends for nearly ten years; nearly everybody in that social group had lived there at some point. It was a real celebration, brimming with nostalgia, sentimentality and, of course, plenty of alcohol. The perfect way to celebrate the end of an era. The temptation to get carried away was potent, but with my mind the way it was lately, I decided I might not be so forgiving of myself if I indulged too much, so I took it easy and was impressed at my ability to do so.

The next morning, with only a suggestion of a headache, I crept through the familiar detritus of empty beer cans and sleeping bodies in my old living room, grabbed my pack and left Ditchling Rise for the last time. I felt a wave of melancholy as my train pulled away from Brighton station; it might not be the same if and when I returned.

My train pulled into Kendal six hours later and I set up camp in Barrowfield wood, just outside town, and fell asleep listening to what had become my new favourite sound – rain bouncing off my tent.

16

Kirk's visit and the trip to Brighton had settled me a bit and had stopped my mind from going in on itself at what I recognized as a critical point. My life had become a series of fairly extreme, pivotal moments since running the marathon, with each event commanding an appropriately big emotional response. It felt like everything had stacked up, to a point where I'd felt slightly overloaded by it all, and in the end something familiar and a short break from it all was what I'd needed to feel, on my first day back, reset and ready to push on. But while a quick break had done me some good in the short term, I could sense familiar, unwelcome feelings returning. It felt like, whatever I was doing with my life, stress and overwhelm were destined to track me down. Things would pile up, emotions would reach critical mass, and then I would run in the opposite direction. It was a realization I didn't like, one I didn't want to accept. I was beginning to feel at war with myself again, losing confidence in recent realizations and becoming unsure how I felt about anything. The fog wasn't visible yet, but I sensed it was there, in the distance, creeping towards me. Colours were fading. And the inner voice, the inner voice that had tormented me every second I was in east London, the voice that I hadn't heard for nearly a year, was calling me.

From Kendal I walked to Lake Windermere, then Ambleside, and from there spent six days covering the fifty-odd miles of the Cumbria Way to Carlisle. The beauty of the Lake

District, I'm sad to say, was lost on me. I trudged numbly through some of England's most majestic backdrops – the Langstrath Valley, the Lonscale Crags between Blencathra, Lonscale Fell and Skiddaw, over the High Pike of Caldbeck Fells – settings that hold so much beauty and character, so much history, and yet I felt so depressed I couldn't enjoy any of it. When my mood dips like this, the world looks slightly different, but it doesn't disappear. It's me who disappears. I see and think about all the same things – where I am, the people I know, my past, my present, my future – but I see it all so differently. Some days I feel it's a privilege to be doing this walk; others, it just seems like drudgery.

From Carlisle I headed west to walk Hadrian's Wall Path, but after doing half of it my energy levels had dropped and my progress felt sluggish and unsatisfying, so I decided to hitchhike to Newcastle to stay with my friend Tony for a few days.

There, I slipped back into a destructive 'coping' strategy of using alcohol and drugs to try to mask my sadness, which invariably ends up tipping me over into a dark place. I became low and withdrawn and my energy levels fell to nothing. I found myself looking at prices for train tickets to Brighton and Essex. I'd had enough. I felt so far away from everyone, from everything. I needed to talk. I felt I needed to get a lot of stuff out.

I had a second night on the 'toon' with Tony and, by chance, ended up meeting his neighbour, Vickie. She was about five foot tall and had a deep, kind smile that made her face glow. She looked to be in her early forties, but still had the playful energy of a twenty-one-year-old. She seemed fascinated by my walk, and perhaps reading my face accurately, asked me gingerly how it was going. In a moment of honesty, I told her that I didn't know if I was going to be able to carry on, that I was emotional and lonely, and the thought of going to Scotland to launch that part of the adventure seemed almost futile. Vickie looked at me sympathetically, gave me a hug then looked me dead in the eyes and said to me, 'You have to keep going.' *Keep going.* Something about the way she said it took me back to the Race to the Stones. *Keep going. That's all you have to do. Keep going.* Vickie doesn't know it, but with those words, she may well have saved the whole trip.

The following day, feeling a bit more positive, I asked Tony if he'd mind carting my pack nine miles to Tynemouth. I felt like running there and working up a sweat would do the trick. And it did. When I got to Tynemouth I breathed the sea air deep into my lungs. It felt good to be back on the coast. Maybe my route had affected my mood? The Pennine Way, the Lake District, Hadrian's Wall . . . they were all inland. Once more, I felt the healing power of the coast and, although I was still far from my best, before the sun had gone down I was back on the coastal path, walking through Whitley Bay, past Seaton Sluice and almost into Blyth.

The beaches along that coast are some of the best in Britain – although I'm not actually allowed to say that. The people of Northumberland like to keep quiet about their spectacular coastline, and it's easy to see why. In the south-east, the beaches are awash with burger vans, tacky bars and plastic bottles, but in Northumberland they seemed to be keeping theirs free of too much trash, in every sense. As I continued north over the next few days, the sea to my right, I felt a calm wash over me, a sense that I was back on course and, crucially, one of relief that I hadn't given up and gone home.

Most nights I camped near the coast; I even treated myself to a beach camp every now and then. Waking up to the sound of waves gently lapping the shore is about as calming a way to wake up as I've ever experienced. Pair that with a gentle paddle before you set off for a long day's walk and you've got yourself a perfect morning, weather permitting. I was revelling in it, and by the time I reached and set off on the Northumberland coastal path I was feeling a lot more like myself. I'd rediscovered my sense of wonder and adventure, and I had the allure and calm magnificence of the Northumberland coast to thank for it.

Further north, as I passed the castle ruins of Dunstanburgh and Warkworth, I felt that my energy had almost completely returned; I enjoyed the golden sand beaches of Alnwick, Boulmer, Newton-by-the-Sea and, eventually, Bamburgh so much, by the time I reached England's most northerly town, Berwick-upon-Tweed, I was back to loving my lifestyle and feeling good again. Really good.

I try not to be too dogmatic when it comes to dishing out advice, as everyone has their own way of reacting to life and to what's going on in themselves and all the rest of it, but one thing I will say is you simply cannot deny the link between being close to the sea and feeling your mood elevated. I was having such a wretched time until the day I rejoined the coast, and as those days rolled on my happiness grew. Maybe it's what the sea represents to me – something like endless possibilities and the idea of infinite time – or maybe it's just the sound of water. Either way, I know that the coast heals me in a way I don't think I understand but am happy to accept.

The night before I crossed the border into Scotland I found a great spot to camp on top of the old city walls in Berwick-upon-Tweed, but then I started to feel like I might be pushing my luck camping so close to town. I'd had my fingers burnt once before in South Wales and I had a gut feeling that if I pitched up here I'd end up getting hassled, so I checked myself into a hostel.

Despite having a good chat with a chap named Vaughan who recognized me from *Mind over Marathon* and insisted on buying me dinner and paying for my bed too, I didn't enjoy my night there. The room was unbearably stuffy and my bunk was about eight inches too short. But staying in hostels does have its perks: I showered with real, actual water and real, actual soap, and I made full use of the YHA laundry wash-and-dry facilities.

The next morning I was fresh and clean and ready to introduce myself to Scotland. It would be my home for the next two or three months and, like a nervous boyfriend about to meet his future parents-in-law, I felt the need to make a good first impression.

17

Sitting outside the First and Last pub in Burnmouth, sipping whatever single malt whisky the bartender had recommended, I felt ready to take on the world. The feeling of walking from one country to another is a powerful one. I remember experiencing a similar rush of blood after crossing the Severn Bridge into Wales, although that may have had to do with the adrenaline of walking beside six lanes of traffic. It's just not something that happens really, in life, and it's certainly not something I ever dreamed would be possible for me to do. On my first day in Scotland I was so high on life and energy I walked some eighteen miles to Coldingham, where the landlord of the New Inn, noticing my pack, offered me a patch of grass in the beer garden to pitch up.

It had been a perfect first day. I'd traversed the Berwickshire coast, past cliffs called things like 'Horse Head', 'Scout Point' and 'Hairy Ness', through the harbour at Eyemouth, then over more of the rocky coastline, past 'Yellow Craig', finally cutting inland at Coldingham Bay. My body felt tired but my mind was sharp and alert, just like how I felt in the early stages of the walk, taking on the constant inclines and declines of Dorset's Jurassic Coast and loving every mile of it.

The next day I felt recharged and set off before 8 a.m., sticking rigidly to the coast, past the stunning St Abb's Head and through the desolate Coldingham moors towards Dunbar. When I got to Pease Bay, a small beach in a cove at the far end of a holiday park just outside Cockburnspath, I stopped to have a cup of tea and charge my phone before wandering down to the waterfront. I found a patch of grass just off the beach, pitched my tent then went to the restaurant area of the park to grab some dinner. At ten o'clock, right when I was thinking about turning in, a member of staff came up to me. He wore a white shirt and black trousers and, from the look of the rest of the staff, I wasn't sure he was obliged to. He asked if it was my tent down by the beach.

'It is,' I said.

'I'm afraid camping isn't permitted here. You're going to have to move it,' he said, almost smugly.

I did my best to argue my case, tried to tell him that I'd walked there from Brighton, that I was raising money for charity, that I was famous (just kidding), but no amount of explaining was good enough. I'd have to pack up the Toad and move on. As fortune had it, though, an older chap at the bar had heard the exchange and grabbed me. He was a thin man in his sixties, with thick white hair and a slightly hooked nose. His hands were calloused and he wore dark, earthy tones.

'This isn't right, mate,' he said. 'I'm leaving in a minute – I'll give you a lift back to mine. You can camp in my garden.' I went and packed up my stuff and then returned to my good Samaritan. He smiled and beckoned me to follow him, and on our way out he made a point of muttering, low enough to be quite menacing, 'Jobsworth', as we passed the guy who'd told me to move on. I had to smother a laugh when I caught the look on his face – a beautiful cocktail of embarrassment, discomfort and alarm. Delicious.

The following morning he left some toast and coffee outside my tent – with marmalade! *What a gangster.*

And the day went on like that. At a little café called the

Food Hamper in Dunbar where I stopped for lunch, they wouldn't accept any money and waved me off with a paper bag full of scones, on the house. And it didn't stop there. Dunbar signified the end, for now at least, of the coastal section of the John Muir Way. I followed it another five or so miles inland, as far as East Linton, where I took out my map to find somewhere to camp. A woman in her late fifties with very short grey hair, a kind, rosy face and the physique of someone who has been active most of their life – a runner, or a cyclist maybe – asked me if I was lost, and ended up offering me a bed for the night.

Her name was Barbel and she was originally from Austria. I felt very relaxed walking to her house; it reminded me of how I'd felt walking back to Robbie's place in Corfe Castle the previous summer – like I was about to spend an evening with a long-lost family member. She was so sincere and authentic my nerves didn't budge, but I forced myself not to take things on face value and did a little digging.

'So do you have family?' I asked.

'Yes, my husband and my son and my son's girlfriend are home,' Barbel said.

'And they're not going to mind you turning up after your walk with some stranger who you've told can take the spare room?'

'Not at all. In fact, we put another young man up a few months back. He had cycled to Britain from South Korea and was passing through.'

No way.

'Do you remember his name?'

'Yes, his name was Jun.'

I took out my phone and sent my mum a message, asking her the name of the guy she'd put up who had cycled to Maldon from Korea in the hope of watching a Liverpool match at Anfield earlier in the year. She messaged back immediately: 'Jun.'

When I told Barbel she went nuts, throwing her arms up in disbelief and letting out an almost hysterical yelp. Her reaction really startled me, which seemed to tickle her, and the pair of us laughed, overwhelmed by such an unbelievable coincidence. The same guy. Seriously, what are the chances?

I don't particularly believe in fate, because I don't like the thought of not being in control of my life. However, when something happens where the odds feel impossible, I don't like just chalking it up to coincidence either. I thought meeting Barbel was one of these bizarre and fateful moments, and being unwilling to concede that 'it was just meant to be' or just a coincidence, I found myself tracing my movements back to see if I could pinpoint where the first domino had fallen. What decision had I made, that if I hadn't, would mean I wouldn't have ended up here? And as I cast my mind back, the image that came through strongest, and without thinking too hard about it, was sitting beside the fire in Hetton with Molly.

When we arrived at Barbel's place she couldn't wait to tell her husband. I was expecting him to be slightly flabbergasted by his wife turning up with a vagrant and blurting out an anecdote before even introducing me properly, but he just laughed along. It felt like it might not have been the first time that *week* she'd spontaneously invited a stranger round for dinner. They were a sweet couple, very well suited, and I felt so grateful that I'd bumped into Barbel. I'd got very, very lucky that day.

That night, in my clean, comfy kingsize bed, when I put my head on my pillow Molly again appeared in my thoughts. We had, unexpectedly, re-established contact, so that was maybe why. In a moment of romantic longing I'd mentioned meeting 'someone' in a post on Facebook in the hope she might look me up and see it . . . and it had worked. We'd been exchanging a few sporadic messages since, all very casual, but she had mentioned that she had a work trip to Scotland coming up and dropped a hint that she might, perhaps, want to meet up.

If I was to meet up with her, I had five days to make it to Edinburgh – and around seventy miles to walk. I wasn't going to miss a chance to see her again, but I hadn't wanted to leave the coast. Now, I was almost there, but fatigue had begun to set in.

The day I walked into Edinburgh I was running on fumes, but I'd made it with an evening to spare and, to my good fortune once again, one of my followers on Instagram, Kate, had messaged me a few days earlier offering me a place to stay. Kate, her husband Fraser and their two lads, Callum and Ruairidh, were a wonderfully easygoing family. I could tell Kate and Fraser had got together in school even before they told me, there was such a natural harmony between them, and all four of them.

The following morning, after a long, much-needed sleep, Kate dropped me off in the centre of Edinburgh. My plan was to grab a coffee and wait for Molly to message me, so I slipped into a very handsome-looking café on the corner of George Street and ordered a surprisingly expensive latte – it had been a while since I'd bought anything in a city. A song was playing that I hadn't heard in ages, 'The Only Exception' by Paramore, a band that always reminds me of my old house-mate Jess, one of my favourite people. I messaged her, and then began thinking about the party at Ditchling Rise. All of a sudden I felt like I was a million miles from home. A wave of sadness engulfed me, my eyes filled with tears and I took a deep breath, grabbed my things and left. I didn't get five feet before my eyes welled up to capacity and the lump in my throat was knocking at the back of my teeth. I ducked down the nearest side road and began to sob. I heard footsteps approaching and did my best to calm myself down and wipe the tears from my face.

'Mate, what's wrong?' The kindness in the man's tone was unmistakable.

I couldn't muster a coherent response, and so he just grabbed me, pulled me towards him and forced a tight hug on me. I began to cry again, uncontrollably now. After a good twenty seconds, I'd managed to pull myself together enough to thank him, and told him why I was crying. He looked at me with a haunting familiarity (it gives me chills as I recall it now), hugged me once more and insisted he buy me a coffee. So off we sloped, across the road to a different café, with a patio. While he was ordering I used the time alone to do a bit more crying and when he came back he told me a story I'll remember forever.

His name was Ibrahim, and he'd fled Iraq with a friend with nothing but the clothes they had on. They'd left several years ago after evading capture from soldiers and Ibrahim had been in Scotland nearly two years. That look he'd given me was one of real empathy. He'd been through so much. Almost all of this man's friends back home, about thirty-five of them, he recalled, were dead.

Ibrahim had made his way from Iraq to Turkey. From there, he and his friend had walked, sleeping rough and eating scraps to survive, all the way to the French coast. He, in his words, was one of the 'lucky' ones who then made it across the Channel into Great Britain. This man, whose home was too dangerous for him to go back to, whose child-hood friends were massacred, and whose family are so far away, felt 'lucky' to have the life he now has, so lucky that he stopped to comfort a white English man crying in the street. And he told me why. He said:

'I believe that, sometimes, God throws you in a direction to meet people, and if you recognize that, it will bring a great friendship. When I came here from Iraq, I knew nobody and I found myself alone, crying in the street, just like you, and a stranger came up to me and hugged me. She's now my sister, and we will walk together forever.'

We sat there for a while, discussing fate, and chance: I'd stepped up my pace to get to Edinburgh on that particular day; a certain song had made me reach out to my friend; Ibrahim had never been down this street before today; and, of course, we had both walked thousands of miles and come to this city. And mostly, we both seemed the type to trust in the kindness of strangers, and had, in that exact moment, acted on pure instinct. Sometimes, when worlds collide so perfectly and profoundly as they did that afternoon it's impossible not to feel what Ibrahim referred to as 'the touch of God' – whatever you believe 'God' is. It's these moments that make life not just worth living, but worth fighting for. Ibrahim suggested the two of us hang out the following day. 'Come to my place! Let me cook you some Arabic food!' he said excitedly. We exchanged numbers and arranged to meet in the city centre after he'd finished work. A few minutes later I received a message from Molly – 'Train arrives in 15 mins X' – and so with that, I left the café and headed towards Haymarket station.

With some minutes to myself, I sensed that I was in a new headspace. The sadness had passed and in its place was a feeling of love, and when I saw Molly on the platform, called her name and watched her turn around to face me, I couldn't believe how perfect the situation was. We hugged, and before either of us had the chance to rattle off small talk I put my hands on her shoulders, looked into her eyes and said, 'You won't believe what just happened to me.'

Molly listened intently, her eyes fixed on mine, a strange, excitable smile on her face as I exploded into a skittish, mercurial monologue about fate and coincidence and how everything's connected. She sat there through it all and didn't laugh at me once. I told her about Ibrahim, about Barbel, and about all the other mind-bogglingly perfect moments that had featured in my journey since she and I had met, and how it was all making me feel like everything, the good and the bad, it all mattered. As it all poured out like a slightly clichéd A-level philosophy rant, I realized that I'd finally accepted the concept of fate, because, regardless of how little physical evidence there is for it, at this stage of the walk it was what had got my spirit back. My time in Newcastle had been fraught because of how low I felt in myself, and Tony's neighbour Vickie had helped get me through it, but the happiness I now felt was all to do with feeling like the world was an extraordinary, wondrous, fascinating place, and when I feel like that, it's a sign that I'm doing good.

Molly could only stick around for a couple of hours and, although I didn't want her to leave, in the end it kind of felt right for her to. If our circumstances had been different, I feel certain that our incredible chemistry would have played out beautifully. All those exciting plans you make when you first meet someone who knocks you for six, all that conversation and finding out about each other to come, it just wasn't to be. There was something between us, but the timing was all off and as we parted ways, still not quite sure if we should stay in touch or not, I was once again left wondering what could have been. It had been an emotionally tiring day, after a physically demanding week, and after wandering the streets of Edinburgh in a daze for an hour or so I checked into a hostel and spent the rest of the day in bed.

I met up with Ibrahim the next day, as planned, and we headed over to his flat. I was pleasantly surprised by how together his life seemed after he'd been through so much. He now had refugee status, had got himself set up and was holding down two jobs so that he could live and send money home to his family. He told me all about his country, how beautiful it once was and how the conflict had turned it into 'hell', and how he couldn't understand the hostility he sometimes experiences in Britain. It's one thing watching footage of what's going on in war zones on the news, but hearing a personal account from someone who's been through it was something else. It was important to hear, but it made me angry to think that people who've been through similar situations to Ibrahim, who has exhibited unbelievable physical and emotional strength and gone to extraordinary lengths to escape persecution and death in his own country, can still be demonized in this country. I felt the need to do something, to put Ibrahim's story out there, in the hope that people who have found themselves condemning refugees coming to Britain might read it and start to question their prejudices. After I left, I wrote a blog about him and posted it on Facebook. It got the biggest response from a post since the walk began, and the outpouring of love and support for Ibrahim moved him deeply.

That night I stayed in the hostel again. I felt like I was in a good place, and I was feeling positive about the road ahead. As I looked at the map, and went over the options of getting from Edinburgh over to Glasgow, I got excited and made a decision. With this new lease of life, I decided that the time had come to start running.

18

The run route from Edinburgh to Glasgow was simple to plan. It was a straight twenty-five miles from Edinburgh to Falkirk along the Union towpath, then a further twenty-one miles from Falkirk to Glasgow via the Forth and Clyde canal path – a three-day, fifty-mile journey with one change. It was the first time I'd ever run a distance of over ten miles on consecutive days, and as tempted as I was to do the whole lot in one, I remembered that, although getting to the end of Race to the Stones was an incredible feeling, the vast majority of it sucked. As I hoped they would be, my legs were cut out for it, and in the end the run was surprisingly easy (it was flat the whole way) and when I got to Glasgow I felt like I could have kept going if I'd wanted to. It made me confident that, at some point, running a larger section of my route could be an option.

The only issue was my rucksack, which I'd left behind in a locker in Edinburgh. I'd have to jump on a train back there to pick it up, then cart it across to Glasgow again before heading north, which seemed a big hassle, and something to think about if I did want to try running again. I was chuffed I'd done it, though, and on the night I arrived in Glasgow I was in the mood to celebrate.

I met up with Patti, who, like many others, had got in touch on Instagram a few days previously and offered me a place to stay. I went out with her and her friends for what felt like an absurd number of beverages, and we all piled back to someone's house when the pub closed. Good old Glasgow.

At some point my hosts decided to treat 'the random English bloke' to a few classic Scottish songs. After rattling through some fairly predictable numbers (The Proclaimers was played twice), they played 'Caledonia' by Dougie McLean, a song about feeling homesick. Patti and her friends all sat on the floor with their arms around each other and sang it from start to finish, word perfect. There's a feeling of national pride in Scotland that I apparently find very moving after a night out and a few after-hours cans of Tennants, and that, combined with the song's poignant and relatable lyrics, meant I had to nip off to the bog before the song ended and have a bit of a cry. It would be the last time I could enjoy the spoils of the city for a while, and it felt right to have a wee blowout before I began heading north, towards the Highlands.

Before I headed to Glasgow Central station to meet my brother I stocked up on supplies, swinging by the local Aldi and filling every available space in my pack with bread, bananas, bags of nuts, cans of beans and sweets. Sam was coming out to join me for the third time. Unlike in the Sussex Downs, when my adventure was just beginning, Sam and I enjoyed a much more organized and picturesque time on the West Highland Way, a ninety-six-mile national trail that begins in Milngavie, six miles or so north of Glasgow city centre.

We traversed fifteen miles of lowlands, woods and undulating foothills to Balmaha, a small village on the eastern shore of Loch Lomond. From there we followed the trail north, hugging the loch for ten miles or so, passing through the Rowardennan Forest, where thousands of Scots pines stand tall like spears and the air is awash with the comforting scent of pine needles. It reminded us of the smell on Mum's boat at Christmas. At the foot of the loch's eastern banks we connected with the last section of road out of

Glasgow, and Sam hitchhiked back. I was gutted to be losing him so soon; his unique energy never fails to lift me and, after what had been a few weeks of mental ups and downs, facing more time alone was slightly daunting.

I checked into a bunkhouse by the loch. Most of the other places I'd earmarked were camping grounds, but this place was cheap, and in the woods, and not at all like the soulless YHAs and city hostels I'd stayed in. After dropping my stuff off I went back to the loch, to an old, rickety pontoon fifty yards or so north of the bunkhouse, stripped to my boxers and dived into the water. The cold hit me like a slap to the face as I plunged deep into complete darkness. The water was as black as oil, and when I opened my eyes under the water and looked below me it looked like I was floating over a cavernous abyss, a chasm of pitch black capable of swallowing a mountain. It scared me, but I felt my eyes widen and my muscles clench instinctively and I carried on staring down, allowing terror to engulf me like a wave.

My relationship with 'controlled' fear dates back to my childhood. When I was about nine my dad bought me one of those didactic 'Complete Guide to Cinema' books, full of stills from old movies, illustrations of film reels and popcorn, and headings like 'How It All Began' and 'Broadway on Screen'. I loved it, especially the horror section, with its pictures (and my first sightings) of characters like Nosferatu, Freddy Krueger and Michael Myers. I loved how looking at them made me feel – frightened and creeped out, but not in any real danger, like all I had to do if I didn't want Freddy's eyes on me anymore was to close him inside the book and put my football-sticker album on top of it. My dad, noticing my attraction to horror, used to guide me through the plots of some of the old classics, almost like he was telling me bedtime stories. This inevitably led to me begging my parents to rent *The Evil Dead*, and on my eleventh birthday they caved and agreed to let me and my friends watch it at a sleepover. At the time, the only things me and my friends did were play football, ride around on our bikes and go round to the Watkinses' (the kids with the biggest house in our neighbourhood) to play Mario Kart and jump on their trampoline, so my suggestion that we spend my birthday sitting in the dark watching an eighties horror film was a little left field. None of them seemed half as excited about it as me. Not that that bothered me much. I just wanted the gore, and I got it. Christ did I get it. As I sat cross-legged on the floor in front of the tiny TV/VHS combo in my and Sam's bedroom watching Bruce Campbell gouge green spooge out of the eyes of his possessed friend I remember the feeling of being frozen stiff, paralysed by fear, but refusing to look away because I also felt completely out of harm's way. It was like I'd managed to extract the rush of adrenaline I got when I fell off my bike – which I also kind of liked – without having to have the accident.

My love of horror and fascination with 'controlled' fear developed in my teens and early twenties, not in an obsessive, serial-killer way, more in a way that kept me stimulated, able to feel the hot prickliness of fight or flight without ever being in real danger, getting high off the adrenaline. As I got older and began to encounter real-life fight-or-flight situations more and more, scaring myself became more like an unconscious training exercise, a way for my body to practise its response to being in tense or unsafe situations (which happens quite frequently when your job is to keep a room full of drunk adults from getting too rowdy and fighting each other). I guess this all came from realizing that real-life conflict makes me freeze, so if there's ever a chance to 'practise' being in a frightening situation, my instinct is to value it, and take it. That's why, as I hung there, weightless beneath the surface of the water, I ignored my body's cry to 'get the hell out of there' and embraced the churning in my stomach and the blood rushing behind my ears until I ran out of air and kicked up to the surface.

It took a long moment for my heart to stop racing. Once I'd recalibrated I looked around me. Across the loch, above the western banks, stood a vast coniferous forest, its colours dark like avocado skin, covering up the base of a colossal swell in the land that climbed and climbed until it touched the sky. My eyes followed the top of the ridge and I watched the swell dip and then drop in front of another, then I gazed across the length of the loch into the distance, where all there was to see for miles and miles between the water and the sky were rolling mountains, glowing glaucous blue like grapes. It didn't look real; it was too picturesque to be real. It was the most beautiful thing I had ever seen.

As I lay in my bunk that evening, shacked up with three other hikers in a room that smelt like dry mud, damp leaves and body odour, I received an unexpected message from Molly. It had only been a few days since we'd spoken about breaking contact, and seeing her name pop up on my screen after such a short space of time threw me and tied a tiny knot in my stomach. She asked where I was. I sent her a picture I'd taken from the pontoon after my swim, along with a screenshot from my OS app that showed my exact location. She messaged back, asking if the mountain on the other side of the water was a 'Munro', a term I didn't know. 'I don't know,' I wrote, not sure what else to say. I clicked send and locked my screen. I was so tired, and messaging Molly was demanding a lot more energy than I had. I closed my eyes, feeling myself about to drift off, and my phone buzzed again, startling me, the light from the screen shining right on to my face.

'You're right next to Ben Lomond! That's a Munro! You should bag it tomorrow morning!' I lay there for a few seconds, thinking what I should send back, then gave up and fell asleep.

I woke with a start four hours later. It was 3 a.m. and moonlight was pouring through the open curtains, illuminating my top bunk and the rest of the room with a cold, bluish grey light. I shut the curtains and climbed back up to my bunk, being careful to avoid stepping on any of the soggy rucksacks, coats and boots strewn across the floor, and lay there, wide awake. I opened the message from Molly: 'You're right next to Ben Lomond! That's a Munro! You should bag it tomorrow morning!' I had more energy now, so I did a spot of googling. Fifteen minutes later I excitedly set my alarm, rolled over and went back to sleep.

A Munro is a mountain in Scotland with a height over 3,000 feet, and there are currently 282 of them. I say 'currently' because the list has (somehow) risen and fallen over the years, with the most noteworthy correction occurring in 2009: a routine remeasuring of Sgùrr nan Ceannaichean (Gaelic for 'Peak of the Pedlars') in Wester Ross found it to be a whole metre short of the correct height, and so it was relegated into the amusingly named 'Corbett' category – which gives me cause to ask an obvious question: shouldn't Munros actually be called Barkers? 'Munro bagging' was a term I wasn't familiar with either, before Molly used it; it's a sort of on/off challenge where the aim is to reach the summit of each of Scotland's 282 Munros, which is no doubt a frustratingly uncertain target to hit for those who take their time in completing it, what with the constant remeasuring and reclassifying that seems to go on. Imagine spending your entire life conquering 282 mountains, only to be told that one of them doesn't count, or that there are two more now.

That morning, after learning everything I just told you and getting excited by the prospect of bagging a Munro, I set out to bag my first: Ben Lomond (3,195 feet), before breakfast. I decided I'd wear my running shoes, thinking that when I reached the top it might be fun to run back down the other side. I was out the door at six thirty, leaving my pack at the bunkhouse so I could collect it before midday checkout. The morning air was thick and cool and moisture was evaporating off the loch.

I felt the fresh, damp air fill my lungs as I set off towards Ben Lomond at an easy pace, letting the blood flow through my legs before picking my stride up to a gentle jog. My new shoes felt incredible, as robust and durable as off-road tyres, and as I crunched and splashed my way through the terrain I felt like a pro trail runner on the cover of *Runner's World*. I was so pleased with myself for getting up and out so early and, as often happens when I do, I enjoyed a pleasant sense of vitality as I ran the half-mile or so to the base of the mountain.

As I began my ascent I decided to shift my effort up a gear, maintaining pace as I confronted the mountain with an unexpected rush of determination. Before long my chest was thudding as I drove my feet hard into the rough ground, leaping nimbly from rock to rock and across the deep scars of the mountain, testing myself and pushing the strength in my legs and lungs to their limit. It wasn't long, though, before the incline proved too demanding to maintain my pace and, as my quick, deft footwork reverted to deep, clumsy lunges, I imagined how the seasoned walkers and Munroists (completists) would react at observing such an impetuous approach to a maiden Munro-bagging attempt.

Predictably, after an hour or so, even my lunging had descended into a listless and more manageable potter. As I wheezed my way up a thin track, higher and higher until the clouds were almost within touching distance, I turned my back to pause for air, like I didn't want to let the summit see how much I was struggling. Without thinking about it, I had gained enough height to look down upon much of the land around me, and across the range of mountains that guard it. The view took my breath away. Enormous swells of jagged, uneven land suffused with green and purple, connected for miles like vast armies awaiting orders. The deep, dark bodies of trees in the middle distance stood firm like phalanxes, while the shadowy loch I'd got into yesterday, black like an inkwell, sat still and silent, watched over by the sleeping giants. Whatever it is that makes the colours in Scotland sing in the desolate way they do, it's the land's most defining characteristic for me, an ancient palette that makes every panorama evoke a sense of oppression, the haunting sound of distant bagpipes; promising, enchanting and powerfully iconic.

Moments like these would occur more and more frequently as I moved through Scotland, and while they always left me breathless they also had me longing for companionship, for someone to nudge so I could say, 'Man, look at *that*!' It's nice to have a pleasant memory, something to recall in a future conversation, but it can also serve as a reminder of just how perfect the world can be, and as time moves on and old memories grow faint that person becomes a portal, the only soul alive who can link you back to that beautiful moment.

Once I'd caught my breath I turned on my heel and with renewed determination proceeded, at a more sensible pace, up the track. I was nearing a point where I would soon be able to see beyond the clouds which, until then, had obscured the peak. As I passed into crisp, cool whiteness I was transported back to the bright, vivid green of Pen y Fan. It was the only other time in my life when I had physically walked through clouds, and as I re-entered the space between the land and the sky I remembered the calming effect it had had on me the first time, the otherworldly blankness where it's impossible to see where you're headed, or where you came from.

After a few more minutes I entered a clear pocket between two clouds, and after two hours of sheer elevation I was finally able to catch a glimpse of what, at first sight, appeared to be the summit of Ben Lomond, poking out at a slight angle from behind a cloud. It felt like it had been put there just for me.

That feeling was short-lived, however, as after ten or so more steps I noticed the outline of two figures behind the mist thirty yards or so ahead of me. I felt a pang of discontent, like one minute I'd been playing a fun game on my own and the next the weird kid from next door was poking his annoying face through the fence and asking if he could join in. Strange how much I'd wanted a companion one minute, and how disappointed I was by the sight of humankind the next.

I thought they were coming down at first but as I got closer I could see that they were making the final push to the summit too. They were the only people I'd seen that morning, and I was pretty sure I was the first they would encounter too. It was a man and woman, middle-aged, both in good shape. They looked tanned and had the air of a couple who were maybe renovating a small sailing boat, or an old, rusty Range Rover. Career voyagers. They were moving slightly slower than I was, the man a few paces ahead, but they both appeared to be going strong. They seemed intently focused on the trail ahead, so much so that when I called a cheery 'Good morning!' as I caught up to them it startled the woman so much she spun around and almost lost her footing. The shock only lasted a second, and then she smiled at me with her entire face, the type of smile that only the kindest of people seem able to do. The man had also turned around, and flashed the exact same smile at me: all teeth and eyes and crow's feet.

We enjoyed a brief chuckle, but the ascent was becoming hard work and it just wasn't the time to make friends. After several more minutes the couple had faded back into the clouds behind me and as I picked up my pace and made for the tip of rock I'd been heading towards ever since entering the clouds I felt the excitement swell inside me.

A few moments later I'd reached the rock and, using my hands, scrambled up to the peak. As I stood there, victorious, a freezing, boisterous wind lashing me to and fro, the couple caught me up and pointed towards a section of the trail that I somehow hadn't seen. Later on that day I would wonder if I'd have missed the path entirely had it not been pointed out to me and begun my descent without realizing that I hadn't yet reached the summit. Slightly embarrassed, I climbed down from my bogus podium and joined the couple on the *actual* final stretch. As we approached the top I spotted the marker and, as abruptly as if someone had flicked a switch, the wind cut out completely. My hair, which had been whipping my face, fell flat on my neck, my shorts and top stopped flapping, and from feeling like I'd been standing with my ear against a speaker at a Motörhead show a moment previously, the air was now deathly silent, like we had walked so high we were now in outer space. With nothing else to see but the couple, the ground beneath our feet and the infinite whiteness all around us, it felt like we'd entered a gateway to another universe. It was epic.

We all stood quietly, nobody saying a word. I glanced towards the couple, who were nodding together in silent appreciation, and I felt very grateful that I was sharing a moment with people who could happily enjoy a moment's peace without feeling uncomfortable.

'I have to kiss the cairn,' said the woman, and she bounded purposefully towards the monument. When she reached it she bent down and planted a huge, sincere kiss on the rock. Her partner stepped up immediately after her and did the same. As I watched them then turn to face one another, fingers intertwined, the love they shared so real and effortless, it became apparent that I'd stumbled into a hugely important moment for them. I sensed an air of celebration in their warm embrace and as I wandered over to touch the cold brass plate on top of the monument with my palm I took a brief moment to acknowledge what I'd achieved that morning, before turning to them and asking if where they were held some sort of significance for them.

They were a married couple from Lithuania, Eric and Muriel, probably in their mid-fifties, but looking ten years younger. Muriel told me that by reaching the summit of Ben Lomond that morning they had completed their goal of conquering all of Scotland's 282 Munros and becoming Munroists, a feat that had taken them nineteen years.

The concept of 'physical achievement' was something I'd come to really value since I ran the London Marathon. Seeing what my body was capable of, pushing it to its limit on occasion, had given me a type of confidence in myself that had, in some part at least, stopped me comparing myself to other people quite as much. Having played a lot of competitive sport in my childhood and adolescence, exercise had always been about winning, but running the marathon, completing the Race to the Stones, climbing mountains, these were all physical activities where there were only winners, no losers. Achieving these things had made me believe in myself, made me feel strong. When I'm depressed I feel unbearably weak, and in that weakness I allow the voice in my head that tells me I'm not good enough to torment me until my confidence wears down to nothing. Reaching the top of a mountain gave me the opposite feeling.

As I stood at the peak of Ben Lomond with Eric and Muriel, heart still beating hard from the ascent, I couldn't help but think of what I could do next. I was only a few days' walk away from Ben Nevis, the highest mountain in Britain, so I thought, while simply moseying past a lot of the peaks on the way might feel like an opportunity wasted at the time, conquering the biggest of all would be really something. I turned my attention back to Eric and Muriel, who had brought champagne to mark the occasion. Eric poured Muriel and himself a glass and toasted their success over the cairn. It struck me just how unlikely this situation was – me having just climbed my first-ever Munro, Eric and Muriel having climbed their last, and the three of us reaching the summit at the exact same time. It made the moment extraordinarily perfect, like they were passing the baton on to me. They offered me a swig from the bottle, and the three of us stood at the cairn, talking, laughing and clinking glasses and bottle for fifteen minutes or so, before I decided to leave them to it. They deserved to enjoy the moment they'd been dreaming of for nineteen years without having to put up with some flapping gasbag prattling on about fate and poncing all their champers.

As I began my descent it felt like my coordination, depth perception and assessment of risk were all performing at the top of their game and I found myself running down with the ease and precision of a mountain goat. I felt warm inside, which could well have been the result of the few big swigs of champagne, but with a smile on my face and a story to tell, I just felt incredibly happy, and when I reached the base of the mountain unscathed I felt grateful and amazingly lucky for where my journey had taken me that morning.

I spent the following days traversing the snaking crags and pathways of the West Highland Way. With the exception of the occasional Highland downpour the weather stayed kind, which was good, as my stuff stayed mostly dry, but as I was in the lowlands I did have to contend with the infamous midges buzzing around my head. They were at their worst when I stopped to eat or drink, which meant I stopped less and covered more ground – not a bad thing, considering I still had about a thousand miles of Britain still left to walk.

As ever, the land was bursting with Scottish colour. Intensely green bracken lined each side of the silver rock trail at the edge of Loch Lomond, guiding me into a canvas of heather purple, seaweed green and flaxen yellow, illuminated when the sun peered through the clouds tinting the loch and the mountains. Being so near to the banks of Loch Lomond gave me an unspoilt view of the mountain ranges that stretched towards the horizon ten or so miles ahead of me. Ben Vorlich and Beinn Ime, two of the highest summits on the west side of the loch, were clearly visible as I continued north along the east bank, past the outskirts of Inversnaid and Ardleish. Once again I found myself in awe of the natural splendour of Scotland, the mystifying charm of the land, the air so clean and salubrious that the simple act of breathing made me feel healthier. And while some of the time I was still struggling to manage a tough undercurrent of pessimism, I was able to build a semi-operative dam from my surroundings now and then, either by being mindful of the contiguous trees and plants and wildlife or by partaking in the odd extracurricular physical activity, like taking a late-afternoon swim in the loch.

One morning I opened Spotify to choose some music for the day, and noticed that one of my favourite bands, The Bronx, had released a new album. I decided that what I needed was to go for a long run. I left my tent pitched surreptitiously on the outskirts of Tyndrum, whose combination of coniferous tree borders and feeling of being slightly cut off and supernatural reminded me of *Twin Peaks*.

I queued the album up, hit play and set off. Listening to The Bronx (good-time, high-octane hardcore punk) while I'm running is one of my all-time favourite things to do. It makes me feel like I'm running through a hail of machine-gun fire, too fast and agile for the bullets to hit me. Releasing a new album at a time when I was feeling so alive, it was as if the band knew. My route took me through six miles of stunning mountain pass, through the hills of Argyll and Bute, past the sun-hit mountain of Beinn Dorain, all the way to the next village, Bridge of Orchy. The clouds cast long shadows across the land, like a giant hand in the sky hovering the way it would before swatting a fly. The damp of the morning had formed small, sporadic pools along the trail, making it shimmer like diamonds whenever the clouds parted and straight, heavenly beams shone down. Once again, the distant mountains hummed a soft greyish blue, while the grass plains that connected them sang in pale yellow and dusty green in the bright morning sunlight. The trail was rough with rubble, but my fancy shoes tore effortlessly across the debris, gripping me securely to the surface. I could feel every part of my body working together, propelling me forward like a traction engine, fed by the riotous, high-speed sounds of trashy guitars and crashing drums burning hot in my ears.

After forty-five minutes or so I approached the train station at Bridge of Orchy, resisting the temptation of a sprint finish. Coach Chevy had condemned them while we were discussing what makes a strong marathon finish; he said it was a 'really dumb way to end a race'. So I went the other way, putting Chevy's wise words about 'running smart' into practice, and shifted down a gear, slowing to a leisurely but determined pace as my morning scamper came to a sensible and satisfying end – no aches, no twinges and no gasping for air. I really did feel bulletproof, like nothing could touch me. That run was, hands down, the best run of my life.

I remember thinking that if something as simple as running could make me feel *that* good, there would always be a reason to do it. Not just to run, but to keep going through life. To accept the bad days and carry on living.

This was the moment that I believe I became a runner, for real.

19

I hitched a lift back into Tyndrum, packed up my tent and wandered into the village. My mind felt clear but my legs were a little heavy so I stopped at a local café to fill up on food and charge my phone. I ordered a bowl of carrot soup and sat in the far corner so I could eat it with the last of the bread I'd bought in Glasgow without being seen by the staff. As I slyly bit into my loaf, I realized I was now guilty of doing a lot of the things I used to get really pissed off about when I worked in pubs – bringing in my own food, making one soda and lime last an hour, getting changed in the disabled toilet. I had gradually become the person I used to silently loathe – the ignorant piss-taker ordering a latte during rush periods, the grubby walker in gigantic clodhoppers walking mud everywhere. I was committing at least one egregious pub-etiquette crime a day and when my soup arrived (just as I was plugging my phone into the wall, no less), I caught the waitress looking directly at the half-eaten bloomer poking out of my bag. I pretended not to notice and stared straight ahead, shrinking in my seat as she walked away from my table shaking her head.

I wondered if this experience would make me more forgiving of customers 'taking the piss' in future, if I worked in the industry again. I hadn't thought before about what I would do once all this was over. Would it be straight back to bar work again? Where would I go? Would it be different now that I'd learned, to some extent at least, to ask for help and manage stress better? Before the thought turned into a knot in my stomach, I decided to nip it in the bud. I didn't have to obsess about the future just yet, so I turned my attention back to the present. To be this rational, I had to be still riding the high from the run. I should use that energy, I thought, so I finished my food, left a tip and set off on the day's adventure.

I hitched a lift back to Bridge of Orchy and loaded up my OS app to see if there was an obvious place to try and reach that day that was within sane walking distance. It was still only lunchtime so I could get plenty of walking in. Glen Coe was only another seven or eight miles up the track, and other walkers had told me how beautiful it was there, particularly at sunset, so I made it my afternoon mission to reach the Glencoe Mountain resort before 5 p.m.

After a challenging start, up and over Màm Carraigh, I was rewarded with a stunning view over Loch Tulla, which, if I squinted hard enough, almost looked like an oasis in a desert, sandwiched between miles of grassland scalded by the sun. After a few miles the trail took me through the pass towards Black Mount and it wasn't long before the iconic Munros of Meall a'Bhuiridh and Creise came into view.

I set up camp that evening at the base of Beinn a'Chrùlaiste, just off the old military road. I put the entrance facing out towards the valley, which runs between the most dramatic constellation of mountains I had ever seen. Until that point the mountains had mostly loomed on the horizon as motionless blue swells that could be anything between two and fifty miles away, but from where I stood I could see them up close, powerful and domineering, piercing the clouds, immune to time and climate and the advancement of the human race. They would stand mightily for all eternity, never having to move or bow down or compromise themselves for anything or anyone. Maybe that's why it's easy to become inspired by mountains – their character is made up of traits that many of us wish we could embody.

The sky became a wispy autumnal palette of oranges, yellows and eventually reds as the sun plunged behind the mountain, creating the most epic silhouette. I felt both intimidated and protected by the mountains; if you're close enough, and if you will it, I swear you can hear them breathing – cavernous, ghostly breaths that echo through the sky like whale song. I recalled my first night camping in the Flea on the Monarch's Way, how I'd spent the entire night on edge, wigging out at every little sound outside. And now, I felt at home bedding down in the wildness of the Glen Coe mountains. I was in a good place mentally, able to fully appreciate where I was without fear, worry or despair hanging over me, and as the air around me cooled and night set in I snuggled into my sleeping bag and drifted away, into a deep and peaceful sleep.

Over the following two days I walked the remaining twenty-two miles of the West Highland Way. Despite feeling physically up to it, I decided against doing it all in a day; I wanted to take my time and enjoy the scenery. I walked as far as Kinlochleven on the first day, via the pass between the mountains of Beinn Bheag and Stob Mhic Mhartuin known as 'The Devil's Staircase', a fairly gruelling rise studded with stone slabs and steps to help hikers reach the top. It heads north, away from the glaciated valley wall, in what initially feels like completely the wrong direction. If it hadn't been for the other hikers I'd passed that morning, I'd have been tempted to turn back and walk alongside the highway instead, but after a few reassuring 'Nearly there's and 'Better coming down's, it became clear I was on the correct path, and when I reached the last step my heavy breath was taken away by an exquisite panoramic view.

Though it was dry, the late-September air felt icy as it cascaded through the mountain pass, the strongest blasts forcing me to bury my face inside my coat as I continued north towards Fort William, stopping to camp on the outskirts of Kinlochleven. It's known as 'The Electric Village', as early in the twentieth century it became the first village in the world to have every house connected to electricity, thanks to a hydroelectric facility built in the surrounding hills. A dam, and five miles of pipeline, was constructed after the First World War by British soldiers and German prisoners-of-war to bring more water into the village, as extra power for its aluminium smelter. The 'Devil's Staircase' got its name during the construction of the dam, as the return journey after a day carrying heavy building materials proved too tough for some of the workers, and on the coldest nights the devil was said to have 'claimed his own'.

The next day I passed the western side of the dramatic Grampian Highlands (home to 164 of the Munros, including the almighty Ben Nevis) and after being engulfed by the miles of pine, hazel and birch trees that guard the path through the Glen Nevis forest, I reached Fort William. I had completed the West Highland Way, and the adventure had released me from a sense of hopelessness and filled me with joy, wonder and fortitude.

As a reward, I treated myself to a meal at an Indian restaurant in town. As I sat there, tearing mercilessly through lashings of hot bhuna and an extra-large garlic naan, I opened up the Couchsurfing app, without much hope of finding somewhere at such short notice, but amazingly, within maybe ten minutes, a local teacher named Hayley offered me her spare room.

Hayley's flat overlooked the faraway hills and Corbetts on the other side of Loch Linnhe, a view which, at the time, seemed one of the most picturesque and inspiring in all of Britain. She asked if I was planning on climbing Ben Nevis, and when I said I was she suggested I stay another night, so I knew I'd have a bed to sleep in afterwards too.

The next morning I woke at seven, grabbed my day bag and set off to conquer the jewel in the Munro crown, Ben Nevis. Whichever way you decide to get to Britain's highest mountain from Fort William, there are three or so miles of walking to do before you get there. I decided to go back through the Nevis forest then join the single track to Glen Nevis. The route was spectacular. As with the West Highland Way, occasional breaks in the clouds allowed streams of ethereal light to beam directly on to sections of the landscape, making the colours glow. As I followed the trail through the woods the air once again filled with the Christmassy smell of coniferous trees, and sunlight sprawled over Ben Nevis's neighbouring Corbett, Meall an t-Suidhe, which obscures any sight of Ben Nevis as you approach it from the west side. Under the light of the sun the Corbett glowed an almost incandescent green, emerging from the dull colours of the cloud-covered land that surrounds it. It was like an artist's impression of the Promised Land, a lone mountain singled out by one heavenly ray of light. I continued along the track for another mile or so, feeling weightless without my pack and enjoying the freedom to move my body without it, lighter on my feet. I kept my ears and eyes alert for birdlife, hoping to catch sight of a red kite or a peregrine falcon. I'd seen the occasional bird of prey on the West Highland Way and been doing some rudimentary googling. I felt confident enough now that I could tell my buzzards from my goshawks, my ospreys from my kestrels – and, anyway, there was nobody to correct me if I got it wrong!

Over the past year I'd been taking on steep gradients – the

South West Coast Path, the Pembrokeshire Coast, Snow-donia and the Pennine Way – fairly regularly, so I was confident I wouldn't find this too punishing. My spirits were high and the sun was out again, the clear skies giving me the opportunity to watch the landscape shrink and stretch away into the distance.

At 1,345 metres above sea level, Ben Nevis is a behemoth that dwarfs every inch of land that surrounds it. It's a titan, the collapsed dome of an ancient volcano that tears through the sky and disappears deep into the clouds. I took the 'Pony Track' route, which flanks Meall an t-Suidhe and gave me my first epic view of Ben Nevis as I followed it to a small loch on the mountain's east side nesting almost 600 metres above sea level. After another hour or so the grass gave way to a terrain of grey rocks and stone. It was here that the mountain's vol-canic power hit me. The summit was cold and barren, with an otherworldly fog that enshrouded it and blocked out the sun, but it retained an almost supernatural beauty. As I stood at the top, surrounded in whiteness, I felt almost like I was having a little break from life on Earth.

I felt triumphant afterwards, but keen to get going again. After another night at Hayley's I joined the Great Glen Way, a seventy-eight-mile national trail that cuts diagonally east across the Highlands, hugging the banks of Loch Ness. A guy called Greg, an independent filmmaker from London who had recently been in touch, was going to join me for a few days, and although I didn't know him, or what sort of person he was, I was looking forward to the company. We set off together from Invergarry. It felt a bit odd going on a four-day expedition with someone I hadn't met before, but he seemed pretty nice. I'd imagined he'd be a fairly big and hairy guy with a cameraman pony-tail, but he was actually a young, clean-cut, slightly pale lad with short, thick curly hair. We got into a good routine and his questions and our conversations started delving deeper and deeper. It was a good opportunity for me to revisit and reflect; it was enlightening to deconstruct, analyse and interpret myself in such a long-form way. It allowed me to investigate who I was, what drove me and to think about what it was I felt I needed to be happy.

We walked through miles and miles of enchanting green woodland, the deep midnight-blue of Loch Ness always to our right, stretching out ahead of us, into the distance. The air was so fresh, so clean and unpolluted, and every night we'd gaze up at the stars, inhaling and exhaling deep lungfuls of Highland air. It was great to see the therapeutic power of nature working on Greg; he'd become visibly calmer and more genial as the days went on, which in turn helped my love of the great outdoors return to full strength. Seeing all this wonder through another person's eyes reminded me what a privilege it was to be out there, surrounded by pure nature, and how grateful I was that I lived on an island as beautiful as Britain.

On our final night together, just outside Inverness, I thought over the last few days. It had been almost like a four-day therapy session, and I came to a conclusion. I needed to make a big life change.

Alcohol and other mind-altering substances had been a regular feature of my life for as long as I could remember, and the frequency had ramped up steadily since working in pubs full time. I realized I didn't want to go back to all that. I'd had so much to organize before doing the walk, I hadn't even thought about addressing my willingness to drink and take drugs, so that side of me had bled into the first half of my walk. While there were times when it had felt like fun and 'just part of the adventure', it had been all too easy to fall back into a hedonistic lifestyle in the six months I'd spent in Brighton filming *Mind over Marathon*.

I'd done so much work on myself during the walk, realized what I'd need, going forward, to help manage my mental health better once it was all over, but if I went back to drinking, I wasn't going to have the energy to implement any of it. Being outside, moving, giving myself time and space to process my emotions, had transformed me into the most stable, motivated, confident version of me I could ever remember being, and I knew, in that moment, that this train would derail if I was pissed or hung-over all the time. I owed it to myself, my present and future self, to not let that happen. I wanted to live sober and, in that moment of clarity, deciding to give up drinking was the easiest decision I'd ever made.

The next day we said our goodbyes in Inverness. I'm not sure if Greg ever used anything from those four days in his film, but our time together had given me a lot. And it seemed it had turned on a light for him too, as the following year he flew out to Mexico to spend six months walking 2,650 miles to Canada via the Pacific Crest Trail.

I'd originally planned for Inverness to be the most northerly point of my journey, but when I got there I realized I was only 120 miles away from John o' Groats. I felt it would be a bit of a cop-out to turn back before 'reaching the top' so I started making preparations to spend the next six days running to mainland Britain's most northerly tip.

Sarah, an Inverness local who had been following my journey (she and I would later become dear friends), agreed to store my pack in her garage. With no tent or sleeping bag, I'd have to find somewhere to stay each night. I put an appeal out on social media and, just like when my pack got stolen in

Pembroke, my incredible followers shared and tagged my post to death and within a day I'd had five offers. I was sorted. Now, I just had to do it. A hundred and twenty miles in six days. Bring it.

The road to John o' Groats looked pretty straight on the map, so at least there would be few opportunities to take a wrong turn. I'd worked out my route, taking in the places I'd be staying, and my first destination was Alness, where I'd be staying with Ali, who lived with his partner, David, in a bed and breakfast. At twenty miles, it was a slightly longer run than I would have liked for my first day, but at this point that distance seemed doable.

In reality, however, as with my first day running from Edinburgh to Glasgow, day one proved to be the hardest. I was so excited to be setting off on a new challenge that I completely failed to maintain a sensible running pace, so by the time I reached Alness I was a mess. Too late, I heard a voice in my head. *Twenty miles is never easy, you fool.*

The next day I headed for Tain, some fourteen miles north. I'd chosen the A9 to take me up to John o' Groats; it was surprisingly busy, but in this section a B-road ran more or less parallel to it, so I got to enjoy a couple of hours not having to leap on to the grass verge every time a lorry careered past me. That night I stayed with Charlie, an old friend of my mum and dad's. His house had the feel of a surrealist art studio that's been set up at the back of a fancy-dress shop. His own paintings, sculptures and collections of photographs and oddities engulf the walls and shelves of almost every room, and he has a collection of mannequins that he's dressed, given names and placed in every room in the house. He definitely had an anarchic streak, and had me in tears when he told me about the time he made an enormous pair of 'flying

V' fingers out of wood and held them up at the RAF air-crews who'd been practising manoeuvres over Tain and 'making a fucking racket'.

The next day I ran thirteen miles from Tain to a village just outside Dornoch, where I stayed in the beautifully reno-vated home of Gill and Jim, a couple I'd met in a café in Carlisle back in July. Sadly, they weren't around, but I did have the pleasure of meeting Lynn, who was house-sitting for them. Lynn was one of those people you end up remem-bering forever. Her lust and passion for life were so energizing, and the following morning she took me down to Dornoch, where she insisted we take a barefoot walk along the beach and 'dip a toe' in the sea. One of her self-care go-to's was 'being in cold water', and after a short walk down the beach she de-robed and swam in the freezing Highland sea. When she came out she looked so blissfully content I kind of wished I'd had the bottle to go in with her.

That day I ran fifteen miles to the town of Brora and slept in a summer house belonging to someone called Isla, who I bonded with the next morning over our shared love of hik-ing. The next two days I ran well. I kind of had to, to be honest: 26.6 miles to Dunbeath on one day, and a twenty-miler to Wick on the second. That stretch was great fun – I'd got a bit caught up in the brouhaha of the New York Mara-thon on social media that morning and had decided to run to John o' Groats as if it were a race – no breaks. I made it there in three hours.

And so to the final day: Wick to John o' Groats. At just over sixteen miles, it was far from pedestrian, but with the sun out again and the end in my sights, the day went by in a flash. I found myself thinking about all kinds of stuff, but mostly about the fact that once I'd got to John o' Groats, then that would be it: no more land. Of all the hundreds of times people had made the comparison, my arrival at the northern tip of the British mainland would be my most Forrest Gump moment to date. When I saw the sign there I shed my day-pack, threw my hat into the air and let out an annoyingly loud 'Woo!' (or something to that effect). After that jubilant moment I felt a real sense of calm and, gazing out to sea, the islands of Stroma and Muckle Skerry both visible, I enjoyed having the moment to myself.

That evening as I lay in bed I got a message from Isla telling me to go outside and look at the sky. I strolled down to the waterfront, leaving the orange haze of the street lamps behind, and saw a faint grey band emblazoned across the sky directly overhead. The stars peeked out – and then I saw it. Patches of green light dancing around the band, the unmistakable green glow of the Aurora Borealis, the Northern Lights. It felt like they'd been put there just for me. I ran down to the water's edge and stood gazing out, reliving the past week in my head, and I thanked myself for doing what felt right, what I'd had to do to keep the good feeling going.

20

I was in need of a few rest days now, and I had the perfect reboot in mind. *Mind over Marathon* had been shortlisted for Best Documentary in the Mind Media Awards and the ceremony was to be held in Leicester Square. It would be the first time the 'band' had got together since marathon day and, knowing that this would probably be our *Mind over Marathon* swan song, there was no way I was going to miss it.

I took the National Express from Inverness to London – a seventeen-hour coach ride for seven quid – and the awards ceremony was exactly like I thought it would be: classy, thrilling and ball-achingly tedious in equal measure. After an introduction from the man himself, Stephen Fry, Mind ambassador Fearne Cotton presented the awards. *Mind over Marathon* didn't get the prize, but Rhian, Georgie, Steve, Paul, Mel, Claudia, Sam, Sese, Poppy and myself *did* receive the coveted 'Speaking Out' award, and we were all presented with a medal by my old mate Prince Harry. It was great to see my friends again and I hoped that night wouldn't be our final farewell.

Ten hours later I was setting off to resume my walk. The return trip to Inverness, though cheap, was excruciatingly uncomfortable, and by the time I got there I was stiff and irritable. I picked up my pack from Sarah the next day, and the day after that I started out for Aviemore, where I'd arranged to stay with Simon Clark, a twenty-five-mile stretch that would probably take a couple of days. The morning air was cold on my face as I followed the train tracks south, breaking off occasionally to explore the woods around the Monadhliath Mountains. The woodland is remarkably flat and the pines encircling Beinn a' Bhealaich stand staunch and orderly. I felt they were safeguarding me through this mysterious place, a natural army protecting me from the unknown.

As I passed through Tomatin I noticed that the puddles were beginning to ice over. Winter was settling in, and while the sound of the ground crackling underfoot gave me a vague nostalgic, childlike amusement, the wary grown-up part of me acknowledged that the next few weeks were going to be tough.

Walking in the Highlands during a cold snap is nippy, for sure, but it's fine because you're moving. Camping in low temperatures, however, can be deeply, deeply unpleasant. As soon as you stop walking the cold creeps through your layers like moisture through a sponge. Also, if, like me, you have to remove your gloves before you do anything remotely dextrous, like, say, undoing zips or untangling guy ropes, you can expect to develop a condition that I'm going to call 'Highland Camping Claw'. Thankfully, I still had my self-inflating thermal mattress, which at least offered a precious few spongy inches between me and the frozen ground – quite a lot compared to no spongy inches at all, but even so the cold was still right there, in my *bones*, and trying to get to sleep when you're that cold is a lot more than flesh and blood can stand.

I joined the Speyside Way at a town called Boat of Garten. It meanders through thick shrubs all the way to Aviemore, offers breathtaking views over the surrounding mountains and woodland, and lots of opportunities to 'stop 'n' chat' with walkers and cyclists – always a sign that you are about to re-enter civilization. When I arrived in Aviemore, just before dark, I found a quiet pub, nabbed a table by the fire and had a hot chocolate while I waited for Simon.

It was great to see him. He'd become not just an inspiration to me, but a friend. He wasn't wearing his usual 'adventure runner' get-up but was now sporting a look I'm going to call 'Highland chic' (which I'm sure he'll take huge issue with). His glorious white hair, which poured wildly down around his face like a wreath of gull feathers, was, however, just as I remembered it, and his curiosity and infectious energy were as strong as ever.

Like so many adventure-minded people, Simon carries himself with such confidence; there's a calm, almost playful fearlessness. He never appears to be holding a single measure of worry, which is probably why I enjoy his company so much. I sometimes feel I carry my worries around with me like they're worth a lot to me and that I need to hang on to them. Being in the company of people as carefree as Simon proves that there's another way.

Simon lives about an hour's drive north of Aviemore, and on the way he told me that there was an event that evening at the Universal Hall in Findhorn he was keen to take me to, so after a quick stop at the local chippie we took a drive over there.

In the winter of 1962 the spiritual founders of the 'Findhorn Foundation' sought to create, in their words, an 'experiential learning centre and ecovillage where everyday life is guided by the inner voice of spirit' on an old caravan site at Findhorn Bay. And so was born Findhorn ecovillage. Simon had only briefed me very casually, so when we pulled up at an impressive but eccentric structure in the middle of nowhere, I felt a little unsettled and more than a little unprepared. Where the hell was I? Was this some kind of Highland cult? Would I be indoctrinated and brainwashed or rejected and cast out by robed, beardy men with slack jaws and dilated pupils? Had Simon been secretly sizing me up on the drive over here? Or worse, since we first met?! I knew that tug of anxiety was making me drum the whole thing up dramatically in my mind, but I couldn't stop these overblown suspicions edging in and narrowing my usually open mind.

In the building, my instinct was to locate the exit points and keep my wits about me. We climbed a huge spiral staircase and I could hear passionate, spectral echoes coming from the top floor, the sound of an eager crowd. The event, or ceremony, or whatever it was, had already started, so we had to creak the double doors to the main hall open.

'We have to be quiet,' said Simon as he slinked in, leaving me nothing but a rapidly decreasing crack between the doors to peer through and assess the situation. The room was packed, but I could see that these people posed no threat to me at all. I was relieved and ashamed in equal measure.

A slideshow documenting the construction of the building was being projected on to an enormous screen and an affable old chap was talking, to cheerful murmurs and coos of acknowledgement from the congregation. It turned out he was related to one of the founders of this palpably thriving community, and he talked about how this dedicated and spiritual community had come to be and what they were about. Admittedly, some of the backstory was a little iffy (there was talk of communicating with 'angels', who apparently gave tips on how to grow vegetables), but the group's commitment to their ideals and the growth and development over time of this community had all the trappings of a classic success story, and that level of success is always inspiring to me. And there was that same blend of strength in togetherness and the healing power of community that I'd come to understand a little more when I trained for the marathon, and at Run Dem Crew. The evening climaxed with a woman in a shawl teaching the entire congregation four harmonizing vocal parts of a traditional Buddhist incantation. The timing was a bit of a mess, but the notes and the feeling were there, and it felt like, for a few moments, time stood still.

The following morning I woke up to the sound of Simon pottering about and mumbling in his kitchen. When I joined him I found him sitting silently, wrapped in his duvet, staring out of the window. He looked so deep in thought, almost mournful, I remember thinking. He said he just needed a few minutes to himself in the morning, so I left him to it. It was the first time I'd seen him look vulnerable, and it made me a little sad. I spent the time I was packing up wondering what I could do to bring him out of it.

I asked Simon if he wanted to come with me into the Lairig Ghru pass through the Cairngorm mountains. He didn't take much convincing, and within half an hour he was packing, and had suggested that we take along a friend of his, Rachel.

By the time we arrived in Aviemore it was about midday and already I knew that we'd left it too late to do this thing properly and without any stress. The Lairig Ghru is long, and doing it in one day would have been ambitious enough even if we'd set off at 8 a.m. Saying that, our mood was relaxed when we set off into the woods. The first few miles were flat, and then the incline began; it was two thirty when we approached the entrance to the pass. It was icy and white, but the colour of the sky was turning. An hour later we met a group of hikers coming the other way, who said there was no way we would make it to Braemar in the next six hours. I don't know why we decided to carry on; maybe it was because we'd done most of the ascent, and maybe a bit of arrogance – Simon and I were seasoned adventurers, after all, and the group that we passed, nice as they were, looked more like weekenders.

As we walked the temperature fell – rapidly. I was wearing sensible enough clothes, but Simon and Rachel didn't have quite so many layers. There was no phone reception and I began to feel slightly worried; there was so much ice we were having to walk very slowly so as not to fall and potentially hurt ourselves. I started to think there was no way we would make it to Braemar before midnight, let alone before sundown, and we all fell silent. By six o'clock we had had to put on our head torches, and it was freezing – I mean, really, *really* freezing. Simon fell over and hurt himself, and so did Rachel. We did our best to laugh it off, but I could tell that I wasn't the only one getting nervous.

It went on like this: it grew darker, even colder and more slippery. It was all beginning to unravel, and get quite scary. One of the hikers we'd passed had mentioned that there was a bothy about halfway, so I stopped to look on my map for the tiny square that would give us its location. Even though I didn't have a phone signal I was able to check the GPS, and my heart sank when I saw just how far away we were from Braemar. We'd have to try and find the bothy. I desperately hoped I'd identified the symbol correctly, and that my map-reading had improved: if I hadn't, I could make everything ten times worse.

Slowly, carefully, we walked, and found a small path leading away from the pass. Hopefully, we were on the right track. We came to a bridge, and I figured that must be a good sign, and a little further on I smelt burning firewood. Then we saw the faint glow of light coming from a window. The relief was immense, and not only was it the bothy, but someone else was there and had got a fire going. It turned out two people were there, both, to my amusement, called Dave. We got settled and chatted away, enjoying the company and the warmth from the fire.

I woke up with the morning light, wrapped myself in my sleeping bag and stepped outside. I'd been so caught up in the stress of it all yesterday that I'd kind of forgotten where we were. The snow-capped mountains all around were the most incredible view I'd ever seen, and I woke my friends up so we could share it.

Simon and Rachel had decided to head back to Aviemore rather than coming with me to Braemar; I think that first day had been enough for them. We said our goodbyes when we rejoined the main pass, then parted ways. I was alone again, and as the sun came up and peeked over the mountains it bounced and shimmered off the ice, lighting up the road to Braemar like a runway. In five hours, I'd made it.

Traversing the Lairig Ghru had been the closest I'd come to getting into serious trouble, and in a way that jeopardy seemed to mark a natural end to my hiking adventure. I continued south for a few days, through Glenshee, Perth, Kinross, my pack feeling heavy, the way my legs feel when I'm almost at the end of a race. Edinburgh would turn out to be the start point of the final leg of this huge adventure. And I'd made a huge decision. Hanging out with Simon Clark had lit a fire under me once again, only this time I'd kicked the fire up and let the flames break loose. I was going to run from Edinburgh back home to Brighton.

21

It was Wednesday, 29 November and Edinburgh was lit up like a Christmas tree. Every year the city rolls out an extravagant Christmas market on East Princes Street Gardens, which transforms the city's Gothic main square into a camp winter wonderland. Everywhere I turned there was something for me to spend money on, but my £20 daily budget meant I'd have to miss out. I'd booked a bunk at a hostel and bought pie and mash from Wetherspoons and was left with a meagre three quid that day. While a mulled wine was both tempting and, technically, within budget, I decided the sensible thing to do would be to nip to Tesco and grab some sausage rolls and maybe a banana before checking in at the hostel.

It appeared my decision-making had improved drastically since I'd decided to quit drinking. I'd removed the temptation in basically every situation to have a few pints to 'take the edge off', I was no longer craving cigarettes, I wasn't comfort-eating and craving salty, fried food half as much as I used to and, despite the cold nights camping in the Cairngorms, I was sleeping better than I can ever remember sleeping. This was all very encouraging, especially as I was about to run eight hundred miles (or thereabouts) to Brighton. I needed to take exceptionally good care of myself: to stay hydrated, sleep enough and make sure I was doing lots of stretching and 'listening to my body', as Chevy would say. On the upside, I was also going to be burning between two and three thousand calories every day I was running, so pig-outs were going to be a daily necessity. With my budget, however, I was going to have to be quite smart about what I ate. At the centre of my nutritional Venn diagram had to be a food that was consistently cheap, abundant in volume and had at least some nutritional value. After some deliberation, I eventually concluded that the Pizza Hut all-you-can-eat buffet was the perfect choice. If I 'hit the Hut' regularly (full access to as many carbs as I could eat and a bountiful and nutrition-dense salad bar for seven quid a pop), I'd have all the fuel I needed to keep my engine burning.

At the hostel I lay in my bunk, below a middle-aged man who seemed to be the heaviest breather in Scotland, studying my OS app. I was plotting a route, trying to visualize the run and making a note of the towns and villages I'd be passing through. I'd put out an appeal for accommodation on social media the day before.

APPEAL FOR WINTER DIGS

I'm running from Edinburgh to Brighton, and this week I'll be passing through the following towns/villages:
Cockenzie
North Berwick
Dunbar
Eyemouth
Berwick-upon-Tweed
Alnwick
If anyone lives in or near any of these places, or knows someone who does, and can put me up for a night, please get in touch!
Thanks!
PLEASE SHARE

Within twenty-four hours I'd managed to secure lodgings as far as Alnwick on the Northumberland coast, just shy of a hundred miles south of Edinburgh. I wondered whether my friends back home – kind, principled people who I consider almost the archetype of 'a good human being' – would put up a complete stranger for the night. I wondered what type of person does.

In some ways it felt like everything had been leading to this point – the walk, the people I'd met, the documentary, running. It made sense for me to run home, which is why – despite being an almost unfathomable and formidable task on paper – I was convinced it was going to work.

I'd been listening to a lot of music by Scottish artists since the night I stayed with Patti in Glasgow – Mogwai, Frightened Rabbit, The Jesus and Mary Chain – stuff that I already knew and liked but which seemed to take on another dimension when I listened to it in the country the artist was born in. 'New Birds' by Arab Strap, a kind of spoken-word story about betrayal told from the perspective of a guy in two minds, came on, and for the first time in a while, Molly drifted into my thoughts. I thought about how she would love to be on this part of the journey with me, heading blindly into the unknown. I remembered the second time we'd met, in Edinburgh, and I closed my eyes and imagined her face in the light of the fire. Had I made a mistake? The last time she and I spoke it had felt so final, but would I be disappointed not to see her face at the Palace Pier in two months' time? All those beautiful, serendipitous moments that had happened in the wake of meeting her that evening in Hetton, she was the reason. But was she?

All this time, I'd been seeing our chance meeting as a catalyst for a seemingly endless run of moments and experiences, coincidences and poignant situations that was driving me forward . . . but what if it wasn't? Maybe it was just a chance meeting, and all the experiences that followed were also pure chance. I'd made certain choices, and certain things had come in their wake; maybe we'd both fallen in love with the fantasy of being in love, each eager to get out of our own reality. It was a lightning-bolt connection, but really it was just a moment. The more I thought about it, the more I came to the conclusion that I made my own luck and believed in myself enough to go with the circumstances that came my way. My confidence and self-belief swelled and, just like that, Molly was gone.

The Firth of Forth is the 'mouth' of Britain, funnelling the North Sea into central Scotland as far as Stirling, and it was there that I began the long run home. I felt now how I wished I'd felt back at the Palace Pier when I'd first started my walk – energized, nervous, moved.

Running has become such a valuable tool to managing my mental health, it's now very hard to imagine life without it. Running the London Marathon, and the other events I've taken part in, have given me so much, and transformed me from a tired, depressed individual into a disciplined, moti-vated one. It gave me a hunger to succeed, to push myself hard, and opened the door to a world I didn't even know was there.

I wasn't at all worried now about the physical aspect of the run I was about to do; it was all about giving me some mental space. I'd been walking or running around the UK for 314 days in total, in transit. In that time I'd become connected to my surroundings and had a clear, tangible purpose. That would soon be over and, if I wasn't careful, if I didn't process it all properly and work out how to implement the big life changes I'd discovered I needed, I'd be in real danger of slip-ping back into old habits. The walk would then just become an anecdote, rather than a turning point.

As well as the exercise and being connected to nature, the

other hugely important thing that had got me so far along my journey, both physical and mental, was all the encouragement, gifts and messages of support I'd had online, all the offers of overnight stays – they had given me so much confidence in the goodness of my fellow human beings. The people who helped me didn't do it to benefit themselves, they weren't doing me a favour so I could do them one in return; maybe some people put me up so they had somebody to talk to, but that's OK by me, it's kind of my thing now. I'd learned that by accepting help from strangers I wasn't leaving myself open to be taken advantage of or manipulated but was in fact welcoming the best part of that person to come forward for me, and for themselves. It was slightly ironic that it had taken a solo adventure for me to accept that level of mutual trust and allow myself to feel connected to people.

After a thirteen-mile run east into the city suburbs, my first stop was in Cockenzie, where I stayed with Pam. She reminded me of a couple of my school friends' mums – the type who never stops offering you things to eat. Her house smelt of lemon air freshener and dinner being made.

The path I'd chosen to follow south was the same one I used when I was coming the other way a few months previously: I was going back on the John Muir Way. It's named after the celebrated Scottish-American conservationist and stretches 130 miles from Helensburgh in south-west Scotland to Dunbar in the south-east. I'd join the Berwickshire coast path from Cockburnspath, so I'd be coming out of Scotland the same way I came in – overlooking the sea, all the way to Newcastle. It would be the only section of my route that I'd go through twice, but the beaches were so beautiful it didn't feel like a wasted opportunity.

At the end of day two I was in North Berwick and took a barefoot stroll on Broad Sands beach before meeting up with Bernadette, my host for the night. We'd met before. Simon Clark had put me in touch with her and she'd interviewed me for her radio show. She had natural, surfer-like hair, sparkly blue eyes and a smile that made it impossible not to smile right back. She seemed very centred, and I'd liked her immediately. The flat she shared with her husband, Dave, was lovely, the type of home you could imagine doubling up as an art or photography studio, and after a few hours we headed to a café called Steampunk, in the centre of town. It was a shabby-chic artisan coffee shop with a concrete bar and old bikes mounted on the wall, and we watched a private after-hours screening of *Strawberry or Vanilla*, a short film made by a couple of locals which captured the landscape and personality of the Scottish seashore beautifully through the window of an ice-cream seller. I was so grateful to Bernadette and Dave for making an effort to make my stay with them enjoyable, and as I left the following morning I again thought about the powerful effect simple acts of kindness can have. In a fragmented world, it's nice to be reminded that most people, when given an opportunity, will do something good for someone else. I do think that benevolence and selflessness are at the core of the human condition. To deny our instincts to help those in need is to deny yourself happiness. Nothing makes you feel as good about yourself as putting yourself out to help another human being.

That day I came off the John Muir Way; I wanted to stick as close as I could to the coastline and was hoping to catch some of the locations I'd seen in *Strawberry or Vanilla*, like 'Bass Rock' – a striking, uninhabited island made from volcanic rock that sits three miles off the coast of North Berwick. Its white colouring is the doing (or, more accurately, the 'dodoing') of the 150,000-strong colony of northern gannets that have made the island their home.

When I reached the ruins of Tantallon Castle I noticed my feet were pulsing and, remembering the advice from John in Newquay about letting my feet breathe, I removed my shoes and socks and scrunched the cold grass between my toes, braving the icy sea breeze on my bare skin. It was the first time since I began running that I'd felt some discomfort, and with it some anxiety about the road ahead began to creep in. *What if someone I'd arranged to stay with cancels on me at the last minute? What if one of my stays doesn't work out and I have to leave suddenly?* Simon had insisted I take his bivvy bag, but I wasn't convinced it would be enough to keep me from freezing at night. I only had enough money for maybe ten nights in a hostel, but the run to Brighton was likely to take about two months.

Despite my worries, the next few days were relatively simple. I stayed right on the edge of the mainland, all of my overnight stays worked out, and the unasked-for bonus of a hearty dinner and breakfast gave me some leeway in my finances, so I'd be able to afford the occasional hostel bunk if I got stuck. The terrain had mostly been flat, and I'd ditched the beach at Dunbar in favour of the cycle path that ran alongside the train tracks, so I was able to maintain a consistent pace without having to push myself. By the time I'd reached Cockburnspath I'd clocked up close to sixty miles. However, although I was sticking religiously to my new checklist of yoga every morning and baths every evening and, legs- and back-wise, I felt physically OK, I was beginning to feel fatigued. And this was confirmed when I had an unplanned nap at a lunch stop. Right there, in the middle of the restaurant, I slept upright in my chair for almost two hours. I still had eight or so miles left to run that day, and when I got outside the cold wind slapped me hard, a proper *EastEnders* slap, and in that moment I felt I deserved it for losing so much time.

When I began running again everything felt heavier, and it took me almost three hours to reach Eyemouth. I couldn't believe how physically demanding the run had become, so soon in. My run to John o' Groats had been far more intense in terms of daily mileage, and yet somehow, only a week into *this* run, I was beginning to feel like I was perhaps only a day or two from tapping out. I couldn't help zooming out to see how far I'd run relative to the entire route back to Brighton every time I looked at the map. It felt like I'd barely scratched the surface and I was tired, irritable and not in the mood to meet new people. When I reached Eyemouth and spotted a bed and breakfast, I didn't think twice about checking myself in.

I hadn't really considered how much of my energy was being used by simply being around people. I felt a sort of duty to engage in pretty deep discussions with my hosts, and when I was with them I'd gladly sit for hours and soak up their stories and opinions, but, day after day, it had become quite emotionally taxing. I was beginning to crave the kind of relief you get when you click your front door shut after an intense evening of socializing with work colleagues or a new partner's friends.

I'd also been receiving quite a few messages from people I'd never met who maybe saw me in the documentary, asking me for advice. When I felt I was in a more positive frame of mind – Jake version one – I felt humbled that people had reached out or asked for my advice and would try and help people out. But if I was feeling low, self-doubting and my self-esteem was in the toilet, I'd feel like a charlatan. I felt I couldn't get my brain in gear to offer any sort of advice, that I would fail, which made me really, really dislike myself (Jake version two). It was nothing to do with the person who was telling me their story or asking for help; it was my mindset and where I was, mentally, at that moment.

I realized that saying something really simple like 'Hey, I'm feeling really [blank] at the moment. Are you in the right headspace to go into it with me?' can really benefit the conversation. It's important to establish that you are not pushing too far, that you are respecting boundaries and, most importantly, it helps establish a feeling of appreciation and support.

An evening on my own was just what I needed, a little bit of time away from people in general, and the mental space to process the encounters and conversations I had been part of over the past week. I watched *Blue Planet* in bed, letting David Attenborough's silky voice soothe me into an undisturbed slumber. The following morning I rose early, did my yoga, had a hot shower and a cup of coffee and left the B&B feeling recharged, reset and ready to embark on what was to be my final day in Scotland.

As I ran along the clifftops towards the border, the long grass whipping my legs and the distant sound of waves crashing on the base of the cliffs below, I felt an unexpected pang of sadness. It felt like a huge chapter not just of the walk but of my life was about to close. Scotland had done more than provide an epic backdrop, it had given me a true escape. I'd entered another world, a world with mountains, black water and green lights in the sky, a world where I knew no one and no one knew me, and it had helped me discover a great many things about myself, about life and about humankind. The people I'd met had had a lasting impact on me, so perhaps my sadness was at leaving them.

The clouds above turned pink as the sun dropped and softened all the colours of the field around me – the rocks on the surf turned a deep brown, the water went dark and glistened. A wooden fence with a gate came into view – the border. When I went through that gate I would be back in my home country and the sun would set on my time in Scotland. I stopped and sat on a patch of dry grass beside the trail. I'd fallen in love with Scotland, and a huge part of me didn't want to leave. I grabbed my phone and my headphones from my bag, and as I sat looking out over the North Sea I could think of nothing more fitting than to listen to 'Caledonia', the Dougie MacLean song Patti and her friends had sung to me in Glasgow. The lyrics, so pertinent then, now rung so true it felt like the song had been written specifically for that moment, and as I listened tearfully and reflected on what had happened over the past three months I became the moment I was in, existing inside a future memory.

When the song finished I rose and ran towards the gate. I unclipped the latch and crossed the border, and just like that I was back in England. A smile crept on to my face as I started running. With every step I felt I was now truly on the road home.

22

The following days went by quickly, in a blur. I'd upped my daily mileage, running the twenty miles of coastal path from Berwick to Bamburgh, occasionally jumping off the trail to run along the Northumberland beaches. The sand had hardened in the cold, so it was easy to run on and, apart from the occasional dog and bundled-up dog owner, I often had miles of outstretched beach to myself.

After passing through Alnwick, I crossed the River Coquet on what looked to be a remarkably well-preserved stone bridge to get to Warkworth. It marked a hundred miles since I'd left Edinburgh, so I thought I'd celebrate with lunch. I had a hankering for a bowl of Cullen skink – a thick Scottish chowder-like soup made with smoked haddock, onions and potatoes, and found a café that served it. My running gear got the proprietor, Linda, asking me what I was up to, and she offered me a bed for the night, free of charge. I couldn't believe my luck – I was so grateful to have another evening to myself, in comfort, something I'd come to consider as essential to my mental fitness as getting enough sleep and staying positive.

The temperature had dropped significantly in the past few days and as I ran along the beach on Druridge Bay the next day the air was so cold on my face it actually hurt. When I looked up at the dunes that line the beach perimeter I saw that they were iced over. It was as if the Earth had plunged into a new ice age. It was minus two, and I had a long run ahead of me that day – nineteen miles – but the endorphins had well and truly kicked in and I felt so lucky to be running on the most stunning stretch of beach in northern England.

I bedded down that night in the home of an elderly man called Colin. It was to be my first taste of staying with someone with glaringly different political views to my own.

He'd got in touch on social media. I was slightly wary when I saw his message; it was very short and curt: 'CAN STAY WITH ME IN ASHINGTON IF YOU WANT'. I had a quick stalk of his social media and saw he had recently shared a quote from a right-wing activist with an extreme dislike of Islam. I thought about it for a day or two, desperately hoping that another offer might come, but it didn't. I still felt uneasy; I wasn't sure I felt comfortable staying with someone whose views I opposed so much. But then I thought maybe I was being too judgemental, and I shouldn't be narrow-minded. Maybe I should try to be a bit more Louis Theroux.

From the outside, Colin's place looked a bit neglected and when he opened the door he was holding an agitated tabby cat. Colin was a very thin, tired-looking man. He wore a stained, old hoodie and a similarly ancient pair of jeans.

Inside the house the ceilings were speckled with damp, the paint was peeling away from the walls and the lino flooring was so old and worn and covered in cat hair that you could no longer really see it (probably a good thing). In the corner hung a Union Jack flag.

The cat, Boxer, had calmed down and was now staring at me and purring, inviting me to pet him, and I noticed as Colin put Boxer down that both his arms were covered in bruises and sores. I shouldn't have judged him, I thought; he was clearly in pain.

The first few hours were pleasant enough, and we bonded over talking about my walk – a topic I sensed we could fall back on if things became awkward. Colin had done something really compassionate in allowing me to stay at his house, especially as, although he laughed and joked a lot, he clearly wasn't very happy in life. His eyes were tired and colourless, and I was pretty sure he didn't have much in the way of family and friends, so I did my best to make him feel like I was enjoying his company.

And then the news came on, and a story about immigration and the UK. Colin suddenly became very irritable.

'I've had enough of this,' he said, almost spitting his words. 'The country's been going downhill for years. Every day, I read about these people blowing people up or grooming kids or whatever – it's disgusting! They all need to fuck off back to wherever they came from so this country can go back to the way it used to be – safe and normal.'

I didn't know what to say but came up with: 'I haven't noticed many foreigners in Northumberland.'

After a moment's silence, he said, 'There aren't too many round here, thankfully.'

This was true; the county of Northumberland, according to the council's most recent ethnicity and religion report, is 97.2 per cent white British. I'd noticed that the people who appeared to be the most afraid or disapproving of immigration, or different races and religions in general, tended to be those who lived in almost entirely white British neighbourhoods, and this made me wonder how they'd formed their opinions, and as we talked, slightly heated now, it became clear that Colin's source was the news, and certain newspapers.

He didn't have the counterbalance of having a friendly Polish family living next door, of working with Muslims or his kids going to a cosmopolitan school. I felt kind of sorry for him – we'd had different life experiences and had formed different opinions about the world. He was a man born in a certain place, at a certain time, with certain people and influences around him, he wasn't happy, and everything had twisted together to make him believe that 'brown people' were dangerous, 'woke' people were the enemy, and that he, a born citizen of this country, had been left alone to rot. I managed not to get angry, and tried over the next hour or so to share with him some of my experiences with immigrants, especially Ibrahim.

It was a tough sell and my arguments fell on deaf ears a lot of the time, but at least we were able to discuss polarizing views honestly, and although I'm sure we both had to grit our teeth on more than one occasion, not once did I or he say something intended to shame, rebuke or manipulate the other. We openly disagreed but we didn't throw accusations at each other, and so neither of us got defensive. I was in a rare position to make Colin think, to encourage him to entertain new ideas, maybe even adjust his outlook. Whether I did or not, I'll never know.

The next day I did a straight thirteen-mile run to Newcastle. I stayed at Tony's again for a couple of days to rest up, and of course I popped next door for a hug with the adorable Vickie before I left.

I ran through Gateshead and south via the old Roman road, hopped on to the Weardale Way and followed the trail all the way to Durham, where I stayed with Kendra. She'd been following my progress from the very beginning and sending me supportive messages. After the documentary, I'd done something for Mental Health Awareness Week that I'd dubbed 'Thrive Live', where I challenged my online followers to do one thing a day that made them feel like they weren't just surviving, but thriving. I did things like go running with Chasing Lights (Chevy's running crew) in east London, joined my friend, professional dog-handler Lizzy on a long walk in the Downs, and hired out a studio for the day to drum along to some of my favourite songs. Not many people got involved, but Kendra did, and as a result she had got into Park Runs, something she hadn't had the confidence to do before.

It was great to meet up with her and we spoke a lot about our mental health. I realized I'd been on a slight decline since my stay with Colin. I'd been feeling like my life was a bit silly, like whenever I stopped running someone threw a duvet over my head and laughed when I couldn't shake it off. I was beginning to doubt myself again, asking myself what I was doing with my life – all the things I now recognized as signs that I was in danger of spiralling out. I was feeling aimless, like there was no point to any of what I was doing, but most of all I just felt really fucking tired. I had been running for just over two weeks, and I felt lonely. Depression had come knocking like a friend you've fallen out with who turns up at your house in the middle of the night, wet and cold and needing your help.

Only a few days previously I'd been saying to Vickie how great I was feeling; how motivated I was and how lucky I was to be on this adventure. I'd said I was feeling so good it was making me doubt how real my depression is. Had I just been chalking up the days I'm just in a bit of a bad mood as mental illness? Obviously not, but depression lies, even on the good days. You know when it's February in Britain and it feels like it's been winter for about five years? You forget how warm it gets here in summer. It feels a bit like that. I said to Kendra that being happy sometimes makes me want to reconnect with my depression, if it's away too long. That's going to sound ridiculous to some people, but when depression's always kind of there, there's a part of you that misses it when it's not around.

It's hard to turn your back on something that makes up a big part of who you are. I've learned to appreciate the aspects of my character that are there because I experience depression – understanding, compassion, enjoyment in being alone. Rather than talking to Kendra about it to expel it, I felt I was ready to welcome it in. How long, I couldn't tell – it's never up to me. But I knew I'd be fine.

Christmas was fast approaching, and I was aware that it was going to be kind of rough being away from my family. I could have made arrangements to go home, have a few days with everyone and then catch a train or hitchhike back up, but I wanted the first time I returned to Mum's boat to be after the run was over. I wanted to sit in her living room with the log-burner roaring, taking stock and processing my challenge as a whole, not as something I had to return to. And it wasn't quite a presentless Christmas: Kendra had a gift for me that couldn't have come at a better time – the thickest, comfiest pair of socks I had ever worn – so thick, she said, they even had a tog rating. They were perfect. I was in need of some comfort to weather the storm I felt was coming my way.

The next day, before setting off, I pottered around Durham. I'd clocked up around 175 miles in the previous two weeks, the longest continual distance I'd ever run, and I was beginning to think that maybe I should take things a little slower in the run-up to Christmas. I found a Pizza Hut, and that perked me up. I ate ten slices of doughy-based pizza and filled my salad bowl four times – comfort-eating masquerading as 'fuel for the engine' – so I continued south with a full belly.

I spent two days running twenty-five tarmac miles to Middlesbrough, in north Yorkshire. The endorphins were definitely kicking in and making me feel less miserable, but I still couldn't shake the feeling that what I was doing at this point was kind of . . . pointless. Why had I decided to run this section? Who was I trying to impress? I'd taken in a lot of outside influence since the summer and become inspired by the concept of running, to the point where I'd convinced myself it was my 'calling'. But really all I'd done is run a couple of marathons and been validated for being on a TV programme about running. I felt like there was a part of me who was doing this for the attention and my original reason for doing the walk had become lost somewhere. I felt like a sell-out, only with no money, and it was getting me down.

I decided that for the next few days, and for Christmas, I'd stay away from social media – away from the content and the likes and the validation – and try to reconnect with myself, my mission and nature. A couple of days later I was immersed in the North York Moors, heading south along the Cleveland Way. It was so beautiful, and I found myself ambling rather than running, passing through vast fields of heather and dark, spiralling woods all the way down to Helmsley. I'd spent far too much time in urban surroundings of late, and with the sound of wildlife ringing all around me again, the wind whistling through the trees and the chorus of hundreds of birds, the inner trouble eased off.

I used Simon's bivvy for a couple of nights, to recalibrate and to be alone and away from it all. The first night reminded me of my first night camping on the outskirts of Arundel a year and a half previously, how frightened I'd been and how little I knew about the road ahead of me. Lying in Simon's bivvy now, immersed in trees and with the smell of wet grass all around me, I felt calm and relaxed. That's what nature does best – it feels like the perfect present – so I decided to spend Christmas there, on my own, wandering through the moors. And it *was* perfect.

Over the following days my mood improved, and by the time I got to York I felt I'd found my purpose again. I stayed with a family of four called the Mulrynes; they all had red hair and warm, toothy smiles and had a young guy living with them, a *Big Issue* seller they'd got to know and taken in. Their kindness was amazing.

The journey south from York is a frantic blur of roads, sofas, baths and faces. I barely remember it. My body was more tired than I could ever remember it being and my mind was beginning to unravel slightly. What I do remember is that everyone I stayed with wanted to talk about their mental health and, in almost all cases, some new ground was broken. The feeling of everything coming together was what kept me going, the feeling that everything was happening for a reason and that the energy I and all my hosts were putting into each other was helping us all, and as I moved into southern England I spent all day every day in harmony with the universe, or so I thought. Staying with different people every night was giving me a snapshot into their lives. Everyone had a story, and spending time with such a diverse cross-section of the country was an enlightening and heart-warming experience. It re-affirmed to me the power of human connection, of communication and the importance of human kindness but, overall, it was making me feel like there was something bigger out there, bigger than everyone.

I spent New Year's Eve with my old friend James, who had moved to Nottingham. James is one of my favourite people, and probably the most original person I know. But as great as he is, it's sort of impossible not to describe him without making him sound like a complete maniac. We met while I was running a pub called the Fishbowl in Brighton, five years previously. He was my head chef and, although he was always a real sweetheart socially, his antics when he was alone were pretty eccentric. He once brought a bow and arrow into work and set up a target on the top floor so he could practise when service was quiet. One time I found him in the cellar with night-vision goggles on, trying to hunt mice. The most shocking thing he ever told me, was that he'd once sent a guy his ex-girlfriend had cheated on him with a pig's head in a box of rose petals. As I said, hard to introduce him without making him sound like a nutcase, but he's a dear friend and my stay with him and his wife Miriam was just the dose of familiarity I needed.

I changed course out of Nottingham and headed east towards Norfolk. I'd been feeling a bit unwell for a few days and when I reached Grantham I found myself drowning in sweat and snot. It had been so cold for so long, it was amazing I hadn't become ill sooner, but now it was here I could barely think, let alone run. I'd returned to social media just before New Year and begun documenting my progress again, and after I posted about coming down with a cold I received a message from Grace, inviting me to her home to rest up for a few days.

Grace was a single mother of two. Her daughter Molly was perhaps thirteen and Amber was five. When we arrived Grace ordered me up to bed with a hot chocolate and I slept for almost twenty hours. When I woke and went downstairs the three of them were out, so I helped myself to a cup of tea and spotted Molly and Amber's Christmas lists stuck to the wall.

Molly:

1. A rescue dog
2. A rescue cat/kitten
3. A hoverboard
4. A hoverboard go-kart
5. A camera (my own)

Amber:

1. A chocolate labrador (real)
2. A fish called squiggle (real)
3. Kids amazon fire
4. Barbie and the pink shoes
5. A toy Christmas tree

Although I don't usually appreciate a lot of energy or noise in my 'zone' when I'm tired, there's a real change in energy when kids are around. Everything feels like it's about to become fun. Grace home-schooled Molly and Amber, and the Mulrynes in York did the same with their kids, and I wondered if there was a link between that and being willing to put up a stranger in your home.

After a few days I was feeling a lot better. Grace dropped me at the station and I took the train back to Grantham, eager to get back on the road. I'd got past thinking that I was running home for the benefit of anyone other than myself, and I ran the fifty miles to King's Lynn in four days. When I arrived back on the coast and felt the sea air on my face I got my first sense that the end was near. In just a couple of weeks, this would all be over.

It felt strange trying to visualize life after 'the walk'. What would I do? Would life simply return to normal or would I feel the need to get out and circumnavigate another country? Maybe Ireland? France? America? What would it be like approaching Brighton's Palace Pier in a few weeks' time? I imagined my family waiting for me there – Mum with Reggie, my sister, Frank, and my brother, Sam. Freeman too. Years ago, Mum suggested that, when I was feeling anxious, I should visualize a place where I felt safe and happy and completely at home, then add three people, real or fictional. You had to include one wise person, one protective person and one loving and nurturing person. Picturing the scene at the Palace Pier made me realize just how secure and happy the people in my life make me. Through all the conversations I'd had with the people I'd met, the friendships that had developed and the relationships I'd nurtured from afar, I had learned to accept that people do care about me, and their lives would not be better if I wasn't here. Accepting the parts of me that I always saw as failings, or as things that held me back, had been a huge step forward, and I had realized that, interpersonally as well as physically, I was capable of far more than I had ever given myself credit for.

I'd run almost six hundred miles over the previous month and, despite feeling proud of myself, it felt like exhaustion was creeping in. I was now approaching Suffolk, and as I walked along the high street in Great Yarmouth, surrounded by people and shops and overspilling bins and all the trappings of urban life, I was hit with an unexpected and overwhelming sense of hopelessness. Before I could register what emotions I was feeling, I began to sob, uncontrollably, in the street, and this time there was no Ibrahim to come and rescue me. Rather than attempting to handle it on my own, I decided I needed help and put up a flag. I have a WhatsApp group of friends who were in the *Mind over Marathon* documentary with me. They all know what it's like to feel overwhelmed in this way. Four phone calls from four very excellent people later, I'd calmed down and had even started to feel good about everything that had set me off in the first place. It's so important, calling and talking, and realizing that when people say 'Call me if you want to talk,' they mean it. Talking someone down from a meltdown can not just bring them back to neutral but can leave them feeling good, because it makes them realize they have connections and support.

Talking really can work like magic, and if you find yourself in a desperate situation, I'd encourage you to ask for help. If you don't think you have friends or family to talk to, find the goodness that's out there in the mental-health social media community. There are people who, if you let them, will help eradicate that awful feeling of being a glitch in an otherwise perfect world.

I stuck to the coastal path from Norfolk, down through Lowestoft and into Suffolk. The coast reminded me of home, and in a moment of nostalgic cheek I decided to send an email to Ipswich Town Football Club and tried to blag a ticket to the upcoming Leeds game at Portman Road. I've supported Ipswich ever since my old man first took me to my first game in 1993, and after revealing this in my email and telling them about the walk, someone got back to me and asked if I'd be interested in leading the teams out as guest of honour at the Wolves fixture the following week. I was so excited anyone would think they'd offered me a place in the starting eleven against Norwich.

Even after every incredible experience I'd had over the past year and a half, I still maintain that the day Ipswich beat Barnsley at the play-off final at Wembley in 2000 (the last competitive match ever played at the 'old' Wembley) was the greatest day of my life. I love all the things I associate with football – the excitement of driving up the A12 with my dad and my brother on match day, the buzz of arriving and hearing a full stadium from the street, the moment you find your gate and climb the steps, seeing the pitch and tens of thousands of fans emerge when you reach the top. It's pure magic, even before you get to the uncontrollable euphoria when a goal is scored. Portman Road was so much more than just 'a happy place' when I was a kid, and asking me if I wanted to lead the teams out on match day was the single greatest honour of my life. Better than meeting Prince Harry. *Sorry, Hazza.*

I stayed with my grandad on the eve of the match, as his house is only half an hour's drive from the stadium. I was allowed to bring three people with me, and while I would have loved to have shared the day with my grandad, my dad and my brother, Grandad was the only one of the old gang who could make it. I gave the remaining two seats to my friends Matt (I owed him a favour for arranging a B&B for me in Devon when I had that bout of diarrhoea) and 'Chav' (just because he's a real laugh at football matches). While my three guests made their way to their seats in the lower tier of the Sir Alf Ramsey stand, I was in the tunnel between Wolves captain Conor Coady and Ipswich captain Luke Chambers, losing my mind. Just before the referee signalled everyone to move out I was handed the match ball, and the ten-year-old Jake, who was still in there somewhere, grinned from ear to ear and instinctively pushed the ball on each side to make sure it was pumped up enough for the match. As I walked out of the tunnel and on to the pitch I knew that I was living the one wish ten-year-old Jake would have made. The stadium was alive and singing, and after I reached the halfway line, shook hands with the players and the officials, I waited on the centre spot and watched in awe as the teams took their positions on the field. It had been a dream of mine to see what a football pitch on match day looks like from a player's perspective, and now I'd seen it.

Ipswich lost 0–1 on the day, but I didn't care. It was the single most incredible thing I'd ever done and, bursting with positive energy, I picked up where'd I'd left off and ran twenty-five miles to Maldon in one day. I met Mum on the quayside, visited my old man and my grandparents, then ran through the 214 acres of gorse, heath and coppice that line the Black-water and Chelmer navigation path, all the way to Chelmsford, fourteen miles away. That canal path was where I did most of my 'training' when I was planning my walk around Britain. I would walk Reggie four miles from the locks at Beeleigh to the road at Nounsley, and then turn back, and it would put me on my arse for the rest of the day. Now, I ran that same path non-stop all the way to Chelmsford.

I could hardly take in the change in me. That depressed, out-of-shape man who smoked and took drugs and drank like George Best had become a fitter, happier, soberer, marathon-ing, mountain-climbing, seven-hundred-miles-in-five-weeks-running, fully-fledged adventure athlete. The transformation was extreme, no doubt about it. And after a lifetime of feeling like I could be so much better than I was, of hating who I saw looking back at me when I looked into the mirror, I was finally living up to my potential, and not just liking the person I had become but loving him.

I felt strong, but I was also exhausted – an interesting combination. My body had become so used to the strain of running long distances every day it was now almost doing the work for me – I wasn't getting short of breath or sweaty, I wasn't getting aches or pains; I had gone on to physical auto-pilot, which, if you're running for days and days on end and still have a hundred or so miles left to go, wasn't a bad thing. The exhaustion was happening in my mind. Everything felt very far away, almost like I was watching a computer game. My eyes were heavy, my skin had been battered by cold winds, rain and sun for so long the elasticity seemed to have disappeared, and my cheeks had given up holding on to my face.

I made plans to see my sister, Frank, as I headed west through London, as a little spirit-lifter. She makes me laugh like no one else can, and spending a couple of hours with her at a point where I was beginning to feel weak was just what the doctor ordered. But as I began heading towards Sussex my mind went foggy again. I can't quite recall what was going on in those few days, but I know that I wrote this blog and posted it on Facebook:

As I approach the end . . .

My head's all over the place at the moment, which is why I haven't posted in a while. I'm finding it difficult to zero in on how I feel about my challenge coming to an end; truthfully, a lot of the time I'm sick of it and I just want it to all be over, which is a feeling I didn't expect. It sort of feels like I'm about to finish a race; that part when your body knows it doesn't have much distance left to run and so decides it probably needs to wind down and make everything twice as heavy so you can, you know, really enjoy that last bit.

In relative terms I can kind of understand why my head's gone a bit at this stage, not that knowing that is making the experience any less unsatisfying. I don't know. I guess I was just expecting a bit of a countdown buzz or something, not that I can remember ever having that before. It might just be because I have a cold at the moment. Or it might be that I've spent the past seven weeks running to London from Edinburgh and I'm experiencing an exhaustion that's far more intense than I've ever experienced before. Could well be that.

Time seems to slow down when my days are filled with purposeful goings on (moving, discovering new places, new people, etc.). As habitual as this life feels to me now, the daily process of connecting with people through social media, crashing in spare rooms or on sofas and getting snapshot glimpses into the lives of strangers is a pretty precarious way to live, on paper. Most people I talk to about it can't understand how such an erratic lifestyle can be good for me. This is why it is, though: I feel like I sometimes tap into a better, more relaxed, more focused version of myself when I meet people for the first time; I'm always excited to establish a new connection and finding out who these people are and what they're all about. For some reason, interactions that lack that initial spark have a tendency to make me incredibly self-aware and introverted, like my manner is somehow ruining this person's day, and that often develops into me questioning my substance as a human being (yes, I'm fully aware of how ******** that sounds).

In some ways I think familiar surroundings restore familiar feelings. If I've been in a certain place or around certain people long enough for them to become commonplace, chances are I associate that place or person with feeling low. And that's got nothing to do with individual people or places, it's just how it goes sometimes; even my oldest and most durable relationships feel fragile. I think, in all, the familiarity of the south-east has led to a partial disconnect from the adventure, and the bleakness I associate with this part of the country (purely through remembering how ill I was two years ago) counts a lot for me feeling a little dispirited right now. As many great memories as I have of Essex and London, it'll always be where I broke down.

For now, however, I'm a week away from completing this thing! And in an attempt to give myself a much needed lift as I approach the end, I've decided I need to make this final push feel like a challenge in itself. Tomorrow morning I'll get to Winchester, the start of the South Downs Way. I *was* going to run the trail as far as Lewes then cut down to Brighton, but after studying a map of the trail a few days ago I thought I should probably just do the whole thing and then cut back from Eastbourne. So I'm gonna do that: a hundred miles in five days along one of England's most picturesque trails. Bring it.

On the morning of 12 February 2018, tired but not dispirited after a muddy week in the South Downs, I stood on the seafront at Peacehaven, six miles east of Brighton's Palace Pier, waiting for my friends and family to meet me so I could walk the final miles of my loop of Great Britain with the people I loved. It was a grey and windy morning, but as people began to show up, the air became charged with love, warmth and excitement. With a gang of twenty or so close friends and family in tow, I began walking the final miles, along the base of the white cliffs of Ovingdean, through Brighton Marina and black rock, and eventually on to Madeira Drive.

As we approached the Palace Pier an hour or so later, I saw that a small crowd had formed. I hung back, letting everyone who had walked with me go ahead to join the collective. Mum was the last person to walk on.

'You all right, stinker?' she said.

I couldn't speak. I felt like crying, but I held it in. I wasn't sure what the tears meant, and if they started I wasn't sure they'd stop.

When I didn't answer, Mum pulled me close to her, gave me a quick, tight hug, then handed me Reggie. I held her lead tight as I walked to join everyone. Freeman was there; my brother, Sam; Giles; Robbie from Corfe; Kendra from Durham;

countless other friends and family all there with expectant smiles and home-made 'welcome home' signs. Their presence meant the world to me. Clapping and cheering broke out, and it startled me out of a kind of daydream. Reggie pulled me on and my little sister, Frank, stepped forward from the crowd, put her arms around me and pulled me in tighter than she ever had. As I held her in my arms, I felt like I was home. And just like that, my walk around Great Britain was over.

I want so badly to write that that moment at the Palace Pier felt like a dream, like I was floating and that I would remember it all so clearly forever, but I can't, life just isn't like that. In reality it was just another day, and the next day was another day, and the next, and the next. Life is just a sequence of days, and once that day had passed, it was on to the next – shower in the morning, starting to get hungry, pop to Greggs. And so while I was happy and sad and proud and all the other things I was sporadically throughout that final day, as I hopped off the train at Chelmsford station after two days of celebrating and bumming around Brighton with my mates, all I was thinking about was picking up some hot cross buns, sitting in front of the TV on Mum's boat and eating the entire pack. Because that's how you get through life – accept who you are and what you want, and give yourself more of the things that you know make you feel good. It might sound over-simple, but if you're after one thing that encompasses all the things I learned on my journey, then that's it.

When I got back to Maldon I got off the 31X bus and wandered down the high street, past the bookshop where I'd bought my map a year and a half previously, and down on to the Quay where Mum's boat *Blackbird* is moored. As I opened the door to the wheelhouse I heard Reggie bound down the hallway and come to wait for me at the foot of the steps. I was so happy to see her, her eyes so alert and her tongue hanging out, anticipating something wonderful was about to happen. I stared back at her for a moment, then had a quick look around for her lead. Sure enough, there it was, hanging off the wheel, and as I picked it up Reggie climbed up the steps, jumped up on to the seat and waited patiently for me to clip her in. As we walked back across the gangplank, through the yard and off towards the Prom, I noticed the tide was coming in. I stopped to listen to the water hitting the underside of the boat, and as Reggie pulled me once more, I decided that rather than let her drag me away from the water's edge, I'd let her off the lead and let her run wild on her own. I'd never done that before.

Dear reader,

Thank you for reading this book. As I write this, I'm sitting in the house of my friend Umve, who lives two hours' motor-bike ride out of the city of Kampong Cham, Cambodia. Two months ago my partner Jordan and I decided that we needed new experiences and adventure in our lives so we quit our jobs, cancelled our tenancy agreements, sold or gave away most of our belongings and flew out to Asia to begin a new life. We met Umve while we were working in a hostel owned by a friend of mine on the island of Koh Rong, and it was there, holed up in a room with a view of the jungle, that I finished writing the first draft.

It's been a joy and a privilege to put the story of my walk around Britain on the page, but hard also at times to relive some of the darkest and most precarious times in my life. I guess it's still hard to write about because, as much as I learned about myself during my year circumnavigating the British mainland, as much 'work' as I did on myself in that time and since, no person or situation or experience pro-vided a real 'cure' for the way I still feel sometimes. Even in a new, exciting country with the person I love beside me I still sometimes struggle to feel like I enjoy life, or that I'm worthy of any of it. Depression continues to distort my real-ity and bend my truth in an attempt to draw me away from everything and everyone I love. It's still strong enough to pull me into the same black hole, where it hugs me and com-forts me and tells me that that is where I belong. But where I was once powerless against it, I feel I now have some of the tools I need to manage it a little better, to put a lead on it and let it bark at me, rather than allow it to maul me. I've been able to achieve this by implementing a few things in my daily life that I learned on the walk.

Firstly, I know I have to keep talking. I accept that depression is a part of me now, and I recognize that I have a duty to try and explain, understand and interpret it, even when life's good. Having my vulnerable side 'out there' and learning to accept Jake version two is infinitely easier to live with than trying to mask it from everyone, and I achieve that by continuing to discuss my mental health publicly, and with my friends and family. My relationships are far deeper and more special to me now, because not only does everyone know to check in with me, but I now have a better understanding of the struggles that everyone else lives with too and can do my bit to try and help them. Support is a beautiful thing, whether you're offering it or receiving it, and if there's one thing that being more open against the beast of depression has taught me, it's that there's strength in numbers.

Secondly, I need nature. Nature is like magic. It helps me in so many ways it's hard to write it all down. The main thing, I guess, is that it makes me feel connected to the world in a way I can't achieve in any other way and, sometimes, when I feel like a prisoner to depression, nature sets me free and makes me smile.

Lastly – and this is the most important thing I've learned – I have to be kind to myself. I'm going to have highs and lows forever, I know I am, so when I'm low I have to treat myself with the same love and compassion I would anyone else who feels that way. Depression is hard enough to deal with without giving my inner voice, who's really an inner bully, a megaphone. Sitting under a duvet all day and eating shit food to make myself feel better isn't a sign that I'm failing, it's a sign that I'm comforting, and if I'm going to sit in a black hole, I may as well make it comfortable.

Sam once said to me that 'Everyone [humanity] is on the same team,' and while it's taken me a while to see what he was saying, I now understand it. Life is hard. But it's hard for all of us. None of us has a say in what 'life' is. We were all born into a world that has evolved and grown, a world that has developed its own sets of laws, ideals and systems that we didn't help decide on, and that doesn't suit any of us all the time. While a lot of the progress that human beings have made has helped us, it has also made for a very advanced, very complicated and very nuanced existence that is impossibly difficult to understand, and I believe it is the root cause of a lot of the mental-health struggles we all face. The fact is, life is hard for everybody, and that's why we need to stick together. We need to help each other in order to survive, and while the idea of survival has, thankfully, evolved beyond running from animals so we don't get eaten, modern life has stress, and worries, and anxiety and depression and fear, and when those things pile up and get to you enough that you consider running away, or worse, taking your own life, you may as well be running from a saber-toothed tiger, in my book. Let's recognize that we all feel these things. Let's recognize that problems are more manageable when we approach them as a team. Let's recognize that our collective goal is to survive, and to be happy; and let's recognize that in order to support each other we have to be understanding of our own ways of dealing with life. There's power in numbers. Be excellent to each other. And good luck out there.

Be well,

Jake

Epilogue

During the years I spent as an active mental health advocate I leaned heavily on Facebook, Twitter and Instagram, using them to promote my walk and to create a sense of solidarity between myself and anyone who had, at any time, felt the way I did back in 2016. But I think my openness created a very specific perception of who I am. Social media has a way of doing that. To my mind, the subject of mental health was important, but I began to realize that content was more a frenzied divergence of attitude and opinion than a united force for change. It seemed common for nuance to be wilfully ignored and for any stance that wasn't presented with absolute certainty to be condemned as passive or indicative of a wider problem. I felt pressure to approach the subject in a way that wasn't entirely me, and I succumbed to that pressure on occasion by amplifying the sentimentality or anger behind the points I was trying to make. In a world (or medium) where the loudest voice always gets heard, it pays to embody the thing you're most passionate about or the change you want to see. But my natural voice isn't that loud, and in trying to be heard I felt in danger of painting myself into a corner. I feel like people will always see me as 'the guy who walked around Britain' or a mental health advocate, but when I first met one very special person, she knew none of that.

I'm back living in Brighton now, this time in Kemptown with my partner Jordan, far enough from the centre of town that we're not in the thick of the action, but close enough that we can still run to the grubby bay window in our second-floor flat to catch the occasional amusing drunk altercation from a safe distance. We live a cheerful and balanced life of pancakes, pyjamas, good music and good friends, casual flatulence, sporadic parky sea swims and periodic escapes into the South Downs. The 'slow pyjama pancake morning' has become integral to the start of our weekends since Jord's mum got her a Breville crêpe maker for her birthday, in case you were wondering why pancakes top the list. I met Jord within six weeks of moving back to the Sussex coast – after spending half a year on Mum's boat in Maldon – and since then the two of us have been inseparable.

I first saw her in a café at the bottom of St James's Street where I used to get coffee before my shifts at the beach bar (more about that soon, too). As had quickly become one of my daily routines, I'd bought a coffee and headed out the back of the café to the garden to find somewhere quiet to sit and eat the blueberry Nakd bar I'd snuck in. Jord was already sitting out there with a pot of tea, a book and a jar of what looked to be overnight oats (which she'd also managed to sneak in). She was wearing an exceptionally cute bright pink puffer jacket – an item of clothing not everyone can pull off, I remember thinking – and she also looked a bit like Natalie Portman. After a few exchanged glances and the briefest smile over the top of her book, I sensed that if I was brave enough to strike up a conversation then maybe she might be the sort of person kind enough to chat. I've never been very good at that bit: starting a conversation with someone I fancy. Something about it always feels a bit sleazy, and no amount of reassurances from female friends over the years about how silly that is makes me feel otherwise.

This time, however, I sensed a harmonious energy between us, and a cosy expectant current seemed to be running through us both. What began as a few nervous words about the extortionate price of coffee, resulted in wry observations about the café we were in, a big old chat about life and how we were both living it (Jord was in the middle of writing her MA dissertation on community psychology) and some seriously disarming eye contact. She had the most beautiful and intensely inquisitive hazel eyes, like she was scanning and storing every tiny detail about what I was saying. After a joining of tables and two further rounds of coffee (for me), I suggested we walk to a pub down the road that served vegan food so we could have some lunch. Besides plant-based food, Jordan craved the same things from life that I crave – new experiences, new people, freedom, love, adventure. I found myself holding off from telling her about the walk and the book and all that stuff that day. I was enjoying the specific type of energy we get when spitballing about the things we'd like to do, rather than getting into the things we'd already done. I'd never enjoyed talking to anyone quite as much about the potential for a life well lived, and four months after moving back to Brighton to 'settle down', we had sold all our possessions and bought one-way tickets to Cambodia to begin what at that point we were referring to as a life of total freedom, away from societal pressures and the seriousness of being an adult, to explore, to enjoy life and to really live. Sadly our freedom, as with everyone else's, was no match for a certain virus, which cut our trip short after only five months.

Before any of that happened, I'd got myself a job for the summer working for Simon, a dear friend of mine who had recently acquired an old shipping container, converted it into a bar and set it up on a patch of land east of the Palace Pier. It was just what that end of the Brighton seafront needed. While over the past few decades the area west of the pier has become an established strip of bars, restaurants, art galleries and tasteless tourist attractions, the east side's only real draws were a tired old crazy golf course, the Volk's Railway (miniature in size, slow in speed and running from one featureless section of the beach to another), a zip wire (not exactly the Nemesis Inferno) and Volks – a very loud, sweaty club that never seems to shut. A little further down is Concorde 2, Brighton's premier medium-to-large-sized music venue, which until the beach bar opened was marooned in an area of Brighton that's visited only by those going to see Dream Wife or Bad Manners, or whatever medium-to-large-sized band was playing that week. The bar was made from an old shipping container, with enough room for eight beer taps and two handwritten wooden beer menus that hung clumsily from chains off the open hatches. In the surrounding area was enough space for maybe thirty deckchairs, which I would lovingly position round tables (repurposed wooden cable drum reels) so that patrons could enjoy a view of the sea and wave ironically at tourists aboard the electric railway while they enjoyed a beer. It was a ramshackle jerry-built patch of land with bags of charm and personality, and a selection of locally brewed beers that would have met the standards of even the most discerning and full-bearded connoisseur.

Within a few weeks of opening the bar had become a new favourite spot for residents of Kemptown, down to its seemingly effortless charm and location, and I have to say I loved it every bit as much as the punters. I'd joined the team as a supervisor, which basically meant I was a bartender who also knew how to change kegs and cash up. I never took any work home with me, and I earned enough money to pay my rent and enjoy what was shaping up to be a nice hot summer in Brighton while I worked on the first draft of this here book. Everything was sweet until the manager decided to leave and Simon asked if I could fill in until the end of the summer. I was hesitant to take the job. I'd vowed never to go into hospitality management again after how devastating that step up had been for me before, but after mulling it over I convinced myself that it would be different this time – working for a friend, on the beach, only for a few months – how bad could it be?

Almost immediately life at the beach bar became a lot more stressful – not that that should have come as a surprise. My free and easy summer mornings of pre-work restorative dips in the sea, arranging deckchairs into aesthetically pleasing patterns and daily repartees with whichever cognoscenti were working in the coffee van next door were becoming less and less enjoyable. Every salubrious feature of my (until that point) untroubled mornings was being washed out by the all too familiar back-of-the-mind management worries – who closed down last night? Why's the beer fobbing? Why are *all* those barrels off? What's wrong with the till? Why was the till twenty pounds down? Do we have enough stock for the weekend? What's that doing there? Better get that report sent off soon, etc., etc., et-fucking-c.

It isn't that I found managerial tasks particularly difficult (although staying on top of many things at once isn't exactly my strong suit); it was more that having these things to think about took away the aspects of the job that I was really fond of – meeting people who are there for a good time, having conversations and, in this particular role, getting to doss about on the beach all day. I had no higher objective than to be a beach bum for the summer. I had re-established myself in the city I love, and after tramping around Britain, and putting up with the smell of damp and mould for just over a year, I felt I'd probably earned that privilege. Furthermore, I really wanted to get back to me: Jake, the guy who has friends and goes to the pub and cooks a roast on a Sunday and listens to the *Guardian*'s *Football Weekly* while I do the washing-up – minus the habitual substance misuse and secret depression obviously.

That thing I touched on at the start – painting myself into a corner, allowing myself to be seduced by the validation I was getting on Instagram, receiving a lot of praise and having glitzy opportunities thrown at me off the back of the walk (getting to write this book for one), I wasn't particularly down for much of it. I was grateful for it all, of course, but really all I wanted to do was take the lessons I'd learned about myself walking around Britain and move them back to Brighton, my home from home, so I could get on with my life. However, it wasn't that easy to cut myself loose from all that. There's an amount of responsibility to being a mental health guy, and I realize now that I wasn't as ready to take on that responsibility as fully as other public figures seemed to be.

The thing that was starting to weigh heavily on me was the expectation. When friends or friends of friends reach out to me these days, it's generally not to ask how I am or what I've been up to, it's to speak to me about depression. And I find it difficult to talk about now for the same reason I barely use social media any more – I don't think I've felt depressed (not in the true imposing mental-illness sense of the word anyway) for a few years now. I still get low, and of course I still recognize the value in being able to discuss feeling low, but talking about depression in the same life-or-death way as I did when it was necessary for me to back then doesn't feel right when it's not how I'm feeling right now. There are many, many public figures within the mental health space whose passion and commitment to effect change has been unwavering, and a lot of that has to do with the consistency of their message. It wasn't until a few years after the walk that I realized that, because what had happened to me was more isolated, I wasn't able to shoulder the level of responsibility I saw others take on. I applaud those who can respond to every emotional two a.m. message with genuine heart and avidity, but I couldn't do that and continue the work on myself to stay balanced and happy. It felt healthier to leave my experience in the past.

After a while I stopped checking my messages, I toned down the mental health content and sentimentality of my posts so as not to invite new ones, and eventually I stopped posting altogether. Some might find that a harsh thing to do, and others might even go so far as to say it's neglect of my 'duty' as a mental health advocate, but I felt a moral obligation to step away from 'the mental health conversation'. In all honesty, after going deeper than I ever thought I'd go into the darkest times in my life, I was kind of done, and I felt I no longer had anything authentic to add, and without authenticity an important subject like mental health is in danger of losing its integrity, and without integrity the subject can lose some of its power to effect change. Or maybe I'm just someone who can't stay loud for long. Maybe my passion or drive to effect change comes in waves and right now my tide is out and it's my time to be silent. It's a silence that feels necessary. It feels like a time to quietly contemplate and absorb the openness of others, to use my energy to learn rather than create, and to leave what I said at the time where it is and not agonize over what I should do or say next.

That's why I wanted to get back to a regular life where I work forty hours a week and spend the rest of the time enjoying myself, and that's why I was so annoyed with myself for agreeing to take over the day-to-day running of the beach bar. After a few weeks of being pissed off with things like the till being inexplicably down and the Portaloos being rancid and overflowing, I decided I needed to fuck off to Scotland for a week and reset myself. I asked Jordan if she'd be up for coming with me, to which she excitedly agreed before I'd even had a chance to launch into my love of the Highlands 'mountains for days' spiel.

I booked us some cheap return flights to Glasgow, arranged a hire car and set about plotting a route. I was desperate to revisit some of the places I'd walked through a couple of years earlier – Loch Lomond, Glen Coe, the Great Glen Way – and excited to finally share their beauty with someone. I packed my tent, some walking boots – basically everything I'd packed to walk around Britain with – and within a few days we were off, flying towards my favourite country in Britain. Jordan packed hopelessly – she didn't even have a coat, just a thin little rain mac that she'd stuffed into the side of her bag. She was so cavalier about it that I remember thinking that in terms of underpreparing essential items and not being in the least bit bothered about the impact that may or may not have on our time in Scotland, we were a hundred per cent match. Once we touched down in Glasgow, we hit a few shops (Asda to buy a duvet, Millets for a gas stove and Aldi for three types of cereal), picked up the hire car and hit the road.

On the first day we drove north out of Glasgow into the vast green and purple-grey of the Trossachs. It's amazing how quickly the city disappears and you find yourself in the thick of the moody Scottish wilderness. It took a day to walk it when I was there last with my brother, but considerably less time in our little motor. After a winding drive round the bank of Loch Lomond, with the smell of damp pines in the air, we found a place to park and went for a swim. The water was beyond freezing but I made out I was enjoying it so that Jordan could see the side of me I was eager to show her – the free-spirited outdoorsman side. Granted, she'd eventually see me for the city-and-sofa person I am nine-tenths of the time, but on this our first proper adventure since we had met, it was a matter of absolute necessity that I make myself as attractive to her as possible. With that in mind I got out of the water and claimed that I felt incredible, which was partially true, but it also felt a little like my organs were failing. Jord was more than ready to admit through chattering teeth that she was dying of cold, and laughed freely as she whipped her remaining clothes off, dived into the car and cranked up the heaters. The next order of business, we both agreed, was to pitch the tent and light a fire. We walked into the woods, all dark brown mud and soft damp sticks, and then we climbed the banks of the loch until we came across the most perfect clearing. I set about gathering wood – which wasn't soaked – while Jord tracked down some rocks to contain the fire, and within fifteen minutes the two of us were sat next to a crackling blaze looking out over the loch. The water was still and clear like a mirror, and all of a sudden, despite having felt so stressed with life in Brighton, I didn't have a care in the world.

On day two we continued north. We were heading towards Glen Coe, one of my favourite sections of Scotland that I had passed through on foot during the walk. I remember thinking back then that the road into Glen Coe had to be one of the best drives in Britain, and as we trundled along the smooth desolate tarmac, with a warm buzz coming from the tyres and colossal blue mountains looming on all sides, I decided that I was right. We parked up near a section of the West Highland Way (the trail I had enjoyed so much the last time I was there) and took a walk. I remembered camping at the foot of one of the mountains and feeling like I could hear it breathing. I kept an ear out for the same sound but it was still light out; they can't have been asleep yet.

Retracing some of the West Highland Way made the walk seem like not quite as distant a memory as I thought it would.

I sometimes worry about my memories fading away, but it was nice to know that by simply revisiting a place it could take me back in time. At certain points of the walk, particularly after I'd experienced something or someone momentous, I remember thinking that there was no way I'd ever forget it. But when every day is laced with moments like that, it's scary how much you can forget. If I'd have stayed with a complete stranger at any other time in my life, I'm fairly confident I'd remember their name, their dog's name, what we had for dinner and which drawer in the kitchen they keep their cutlery; whereas after staying with a different person every night, as I did while I ran back home from Edinburgh, I worry that one day I'll barely be able to recall their faces.

On day three we discovered that the Isle of Skye is accessible by road. So after a breakfast of tattie scones and beans at Loch Oich we decided to take advantage and took the long road west. More glorious mountain ranges awaited us, sitting calmly with great authority in the middle and far distance, the wind and rain only adding more Highland romance to a truly extraordinary place. Skye was the only place we visited that I hadn't already seen, and, feeling that the sentence 'When I was on the walk . . .' had featured way too heavily during our trip, it was important that Jord and I saw something new together. As with our first conversation in the café on St James's Street, it was more exciting to me that the two of us were looking forward together, rather than reminiscing about times when we weren't in each other's lives. That's probably a pretty common way of thinking when you're falling in love, as I clearly was. As the days went on and the two of us continued to be enchanted by our surroundings, the more I realized that this could very much be how we spent much of our time – discovering new places, holding on to each other tightly and sharing calm, inspired silences. We'd only been in each other's lives for three months, and already I'd realized that Jordan was all I'd ever wanted from a companion. The door to my future was one I couldn't wait to walk through, as long as she was there to walk through it with me. In the late afternoon we drove east along deserted roads, past Achnasheen, before pitching up just outside Inverness.

On day four we ate breakfast at a windy Dores beach as we took in the eerie grandeur of Loch Ness, before driving south into the Cairngorms. We took a damp, crunchy walk through the woods outside Aviemore, where the pines guarded the walkways just as orderly as they had the last time I was there. That evening we wild-camped a few miles north of Pitlochry, and again, using rocks from a nearby river and wood from an old, abandoned house, we built a fire that kept us warm through the night. Brighton seemed a million miles away.

On our final day we drove slowly through back roads to savour the last bit of the vast and majestic Cairngorms, and in doing so managed to spot some exciting animals; we sat and watched a herd of stags who watched us back, and caught sight of a golden eagle perched on a rock as we continued south. We took a cold swim in Loch Tay as a wee livener before hunkering down just outside Balloch. We made dinner in a near perfect spot with a wide view of the mountains and set an alarm to wake up at sunrise.

After six full days we dropped off the hire car and flew back to Brighton, feeling relaxed, reset and very much in love, and when I arrived back at the beach bar the following day, I was ready to deal with everything. The rest of the summer was everything I wanted it to be.

I do kind of wish I could just pack up my bag and disappear again for six months but realistically I can't do that any more – not in the same way I did before at least. For an adventure to have the same impact on me that my walk around Britain had, I'd probably have to go through an equally horrible time beforehand. That's not something I ever want to go through again. What my little whistle-stop Highland tour with Jord showed me, however, is that I don't need to disappear into the wilderness every time life gets a bit hard; I just need to switch off – so whether that's flying to Scotland, spending a weekend on Mum's boat, heading into the downs or just meeting a good-energy friend for a coffee, finding time to do these sorts of things are what'll keep me from spiralling again. Since my walk around Britain I've thought a lot about how to move forward with my life, and what I've come to realize is that while I now have a better idea of how to balance my mental health, I don't need to be a public mental health person. I've poured so much of myself into this book. It's not just a time capsule; it's a place where my darkest memories and vulnerabilities are stored, and there's catharsis in turning those thoughts into something physical and having them sat on bookshelves forever.

I still believe there's comfort in numbers, and so I hope this book helps those who connect with my story during darker times. It's difficult for me not to feel like I'm done with talking about mental health. I'm not done with it; I think I'm just done dissecting it. And for now I'm enjoying the silence, because at this point I'm doing OK, and all I want is to enjoy my life. I think I'm doing an OK job at that.

Acknowledgements

I must start by thanking my perfect, very small partner, Jordan. From making me get my laptop out when I couldn't be bothered to helping me write sections I wasn't sure I could to leaving me sweets by the computer, she's as much to thank for getting this book finished as I am. I love you, Jords. Thank you for everything x

Next to my wonderful and unique family . . . to Mum and Dad for your constant love and guidance; to Sam, who walked with me more than anyone and who I will always look up to; to Frank, who kept my spirits high and whose unwavering support kept me going even when I felt like giving up; to my Nanoid and Grangus for being the rocks I have needed to succeed in life; to Norman, Grandad, Uncle Paul and Uncle Julien for their slightly more bloke-ish but equally valuable support; to Freeman, who is as much a part of this family as anyone and who I know has always had and will always have my back; and to the rest of my family, who helped fund the walk and cheered me on every step of the way – Lin and Malc; Scott, Nicki and family; Mich, Ollie and family; Aleks, K and Henry; Krissy, Leah and Lois; Marcus; Laura; Claire, Adam, Abe and Ben; Debby; John and Vera; Gaz and V; and finally, Julie and Tim, whose generosity and support during the Coronavirus lockdown has been immeasurable and has categorically helped make this a better book.

I'd also like to thank my friends, starting with the Maldon boys . . . Mike (+Emily, Oz and Orla) for a classic send-off dinner and for being (without question) my number-one YouTube fan; Giles, for bringing your calm and supportive vibes to the summit of Snowdon with me; and Nat, who may be on the other side of the world but never feels that far away to me – you three are my oldest and best friends and always will be. Next to Danny P, James and Chris, who made me feel like Maldon was close by when I was so far away. To my friends who joined me on the road . . . Ads, Casey, Kirk, Si, Bungle, Chav, James W, Lele and Kel, Lang, and anyone else who I might have forgotten who made an appearance and clocked up miles with me. To my friends who checked in on me periodically during the time I was living in a tent . . . Sammy, Phil, Jess, Gaz and Laura, Stu, Matt Steves, Ed B, Gez, Tom, Amelia, Dando, Woody, Hayley, Brodi, Gary (don't suppose you've got a quid for a cup of tea, have you?), Felix, and a special thanks to Emma, who threw an excellent welcome-home knees-up at the Bottom's Rest.

Thank you to my *Mind over Marathon* family, who continue to inspire and support me and one another . . . Charlie, Claudia, Chevy, Sam, Paul, Rhian, Poppy, Mel, Nick, Steve, Sese, Georgie, Pete, Claire, Jordan, Emily, Fi, Robi and the rest of the team. You'll forever have a special place in my heart.

To the people who I met along the way who became friends . . . Toadie, Sarah, Simon, Kenny, Bryony, Robbie, 'Charlie', Kate and Glen, and everyone who either put me up, bought me lunch or stopped me to chat and generally made the walk the enjoyable and characterful experience it was, there are just so many of you I can't even begin to start writing names.

And finally, a huge thank-you to everybody who helped fund the walk and helped raise funds for the Mental Health Foundation . . . .

Glynn, Andreas, Linda, Chandni, Scott, Sue and Rich, Kathryn, Harriet, Leanne, James, Will, Gemma, Matt, Louise, Hannah and Fred, Valerie Wall, Rio, Alex, Peter, Verity, Dave Staffell, Laura, Robin, Emma, Alastair, Steve and Claire,

Brendan, Katie, Vanessa, Gumbo and Heather, Stoner, Gareth, Emily, Jenn, Tamsin, Beale, Kirsty, Carla, Maxine, Mat Harries, Marc and Jess, Holly and the Hallets, Lizzy, Sean, Foxy, Paul L, the Sowerbys, Cav, Phil, Toby, Tessa and Chris, Marcus Z, Dando, Hayley, Jamie, Rob M, Matt E, Chloe, Beth, Jo, Daniel, Mark, Ally, Debby, Katie P, Tannah, Paul, Matt, Phin, Callum, Ria, Sophie, Sophy, Liss, Jenny, Joey, Thom, Kate, Mikaela, Jess, Dan, Sash, Jess, Alison, Ollie B, Carmody, James Stott, Issy Wright, John Harkins, Dan Dice, Sam, Adam Foster, Alex, Elsie, Sam G, Georgina, Bethany, Hampton, Chris and Becky, Chloe Shearman, Gotel, Christie, Fiona, Alice, Rich, Alex, Liam Leeson, Woody, Greenyer, Jason, Margaret, Tyler, Rebecca, James, Kate, Thom Lowe, Reece, Sarah, Dan Roberts, Pam and Hamish, Vicki, Rodders, Dave Staffell, Katy, Owen, Paddy, Ruby, Clark, Kim Russell, Stu Milburn, Adrian Storry, Kt Monk, Jez, Tracey, Karan, Kelli, She, Kelsey, Alice, Carol, Fiona, Abigail, Catherine, Dawn, Richard, Pen, Donna, Polly, Paula Rimmer, Louise, Liina, Joel, Louise, Francesca, Derek, Sian, Josie, Megan, Frances, Claire, Pat, Kevin, Alyx, Robi, Ann, Mark, Amanda, Susie, Carolyn, Terianne, Vivio, Chris, Philippa, Steph, Warren, Liz, Kim, Anna, David Russell, Stu, Claudia, Susan, Mark, Sandy, Christina, Anita, Elaine, Lorna, Joanna, Sally, Kaye, Rachael, Dennis, Lisa, Roy, Beth, Erica, Fredi Threlfall, Karen, Wayne, Nuala, Caryl, Gem, Dominique, Andrew, Wendy, Moe, Naomi, Toni, Alexa, Aisha, Alec, Suzy, Nichola, Heather, Jean, Kirsten, Imogen, Anne-Marie, Karl, Philip, Ian, Peter, Jevans, Sam Walker, Nick Barron, Niband John, Fia Gosling, Dina, Ed, Liz, Ellie, Howard, and all of the 'anonymous' donaters – thank you all so much.

He just wanted a decent book to read ...

Not too much to ask, is it? It was in 1935 when Allen Lane, Managing Director of Bodley Head Publishers, stood on a platform at Exeter railway station looking for something good to read on his journey back to London. His choice was limited to popular magazines and poor-quality paperbacks – the same choice faced every day by the vast majority of readers, few of whom could afford hardbacks. Lane's disappointment and subsequent anger at the range of books generally available led him to found a company – and change the world.

'We believed in the existence in this country of a vast reading public for intelligent books at a low price, and staked everything on it'
Sir Allen Lane, 1902–1970, founder of Penguin Books

The quality paperback had arrived – and not just in bookshops. Lane was adamant that his Penguins should appear in chain stores and tobacconists, and should cost no more than a packet of cigarettes.

   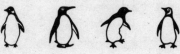

Reading habits (and cigarette prices) have changed since 1935, but Penguin still believes in publishing the best books for everybody to enjoy. We still believe that good design costs no more than bad design, and we still believe that quality books published passionately and responsibly make the world a better place.

So wherever you see the little bird – whether it's on a piece of prize-winning literary fiction or a celebrity autobiography, political tour de force or historical masterpiece, a serial-killer thriller, reference book, world classic or a piece of pure escapism – you can bet that it represents the very best that the genre has to offer.

Whatever you like to read – trust Penguin.